ELECTROCARDIOGRAPHY FOR THE ANAESTHETIST

ELECTROCARDIOGRAPHY FOR THE ANAESTHETIST

BY W. N. ROLLASON

MB MRCS DA FFARCS

Head of Department of Anaesthetics
The Royal Infirmary and University of Aberdeen

WITH A CONTRIBUTION BY
J. M. HOUGH

MA

Department of Physics
University of Hull

AND A FOREWORD BY
WILLIAM W. MUSHIN

CBE MA MB BS FFARCS
(Hon) FFARACS FFARCSI FFA(SA)

Professor of Anaesthetics
Welsh National School of Medicine

FOURTH EDITION

BLACKWELL SCIENTIFIC PUBLICATIONS
OXFORD LONDON EDINBURGH MELBOURNE

© 1964, 1969, 1975, 1980 by
Blackwell Scientific Publications
Editorial offices:
Osney Mead, Oxford, OX2 0EL
8 John Street, London, WC1N 2ES
9 Forrest Road, Edinburgh, EH1 2QH
214 Berkeley Street, Carlton
   Victoria 3053, Australia

First published 1964
Second edition 1969
Third edition 1975
Fourth edition 1980

Set in Monophoto Times by
the Alden Press, Oxford
Printed and bound by
Billing & Sons Ltd
Guildford, London & Worcester

DISTRIBUTORS

USA
   Blackwell Mosby Book Distributors
   11830 Westline Industrial Drive
   St Louis, Missouri 63141

Canada
   Blackwell Mosby Book Distributors
   86 Northline Road, Toronto
   Ontario, M4B 3E5

Australia
   Blackwell Scientific Book
   Distributors
   214 Berkeley Street, Carlton
   Victoria 3053

British Library
Cataloguing in Publication Data

Rollason, William Norman
   Electrocardiography for the anaesthetist.—
   4th ed.
   1. Electrocardiography
   2. Anesthesia
   I. Title
   616.1'2'0754   RC683.5.E5

ISBN 0-632-00543-2

CONTENTS

FOREWORD

If the anaesthetist is to take notice of physiological changes in his patient and to relate his activities to them in a reasonable and flexible manner, he must receive continuous, reliable and quantitative information about these changes. The scientific instrument industry has been sensitive to this need and has responded quickly. There are now available highly developed devices for monitoring the main physiological systems of the body.

The problem facing the anaesthetist is interpretation. The barriers which have grown up round each field of medical knowledge often effectively prevent even basic information and terminology flowing readily from one field to another. It is essential and pressing that these barriers be broken down if the full benefit of the great advances in medical science be available to all who need them.

Electrocardiography is an example of this problem. The display and the recording of the electrical changes within the heart and their interpretation in terms of function and disease, is now widely practised and elaborate instruments to this end are readily available. Interested physicians all over the world devote their lives to a study of this matter and have developed great expertise and interpretive skill. The anaesthetist is realizing to an increasing extent the importance of electrocardiography as a source of information about the action of the heart, but he often lacks the ability to derive the fullest information from the electrocardiogram. As a result the accumulation of knowledge about the effects of anaesthesia on the heart is slow. But, just as the cardiologist will have to learn enough of anaesthesia to understand its relation to his field, and there are many obvious problems linking these two, so will the anaesthetist have to learn enough about cardiology and the electrocardiogram to predict, observe and minimize the harmful effects of his anaesthetics on the heart. This he must be able to do since the need arises in the operating theatre and other places where an expert colleague may not be available for advice.

Dr Rollason sets out to satisfy this need. His book is written by an anaesthetist for anaesthetists. The author does not aim to make his anaesthetist colleagues electrocardiographic experts, nor to displace or disdain the true expert in that field. He does, however, present a simple but accurate introduction to electrocardiography with particular reference to the electrical changes in the heart which occur in the special circumstances of modern anaesthesia. His own studies and contributions concerning electrocardiography during anaesthesia have been considerable. He speaks therefore not only as an anaesthetist, sensitive to the needs of his colleagues, but as one with some claim to expert knowledge of electrocardiography and its interpretation in anaesthesia.

His book will undoubtedly encourage more anaesthetists to use modern physiological monitoring instruments and to learn how to interpret and make use of the information they provide. In time these instruments will be accepted by all as essential aids to safe anaesthesia. Electrocardiography is without question one of the important major examples. In adopting this view and practice, anaesthetists will, while not lessening the content of art, increase enormously that of science, in anaesthesia.

WILLIAM W. MUSHIN

MA, MB, BS, FFARCS,

(HON)FFARACS, FFARCSI, FFA(SA)

Professor of Anaesthetics
Welsh National School of Medicine

PREFACE TO FOURTH EDITION

In this, as in previous editions, an endeavour has been made to incorporate both the developments of the intervening years and the suggestions made by the reviewers of the third edition.

More recent concepts of the electrophysiology and anatomy of the conduction system of the heart have been incorporated into Chapters 1 and 3.

A systematic scrutiny of the preoperative ECG has been added to Chapter 3 and the ECG in cardiac arrest has been considered in more detail in Chapter 6.

In a short monograph it is not possible to be both historic and contemporary. References to some of the classical foundations have been omitted but those interested in them can consult earlier editions.

Obsolete figures have been deleted and more recent ones added. For the preparation of these I am grateful to my son Anthony N. Rollason, MMAA and the Department of Medical Illustration, University of Aberdeen.

I am grateful to my friend, James M. Hough, MA, Department of Physics, University of Hull for his help in the preparation of this edition and for updating Appendix I. I am also grateful to my colleague, James McG. Imray, FFARCS, for updating the section on cardiac surgery in Chapter 5.

My thanks are also due to my daughter, Anne M. Rollason, BEd, for assistance in the preparation of the manuscript and to Mrs A. Anderson for typing it.

Last but not least, I am grateful to the publishers for their cooperation.

Aberdeen, May 1979   W.N. Rollason

PREFACE TO FIRST EDITION

During the past decade the ECG has established itself as an important ancillary aid to the anaesthetist not only during surgery and anaesthesia, under the peculiar conditions of the operating theatre, but also in the pre- and post-operative periods. This aid, however, is only of value if the anaesthetist is capable of interpreting the significance of the changes it portrays.

While there are a number of standard works on electrocardiography, both introductory and comprehensive, available for study, they do not present the subject from the point of view of the anaesthetist, and it is hoped that this small volume may help to remedy this defect. In presenting it an endeavour has been made to steer between the Scylla of over-simplification and inadequate presentation on the one hand, and the Charybdis of complexity and lack of clarity on the other. It is however in no way intended to supplant any of the existing works on the subject, but rather to complement them.

I wish to extend my sincere thanks and appreciation to Dr D.S. Short and Mr J.M. Hough, MA, who reviewed the manuscript and offered many helpful suggestions, which have been incorporated. I am also grateful to Mr Hough for his assistance in writing chapter 6. My grateful thanks are also due to Mr W. Topp for all the reproductions, to my secretary Mrs A.H. Dickson for her unstinting help, and to Professor W.W. Mushin for his generous foreword.

Aberdeen, September 1963   W.N. Rollason

ACKNOWLEDGEMENTS

I am grateful to the following for permission to reproduce the illustrations indicated:

Dr S.R. Arbeit and F.A. Davis Company, Philadelphia for Figs. 19, 20, 21, 26, 28, 38, 39, 42, 45, 51, (from *Differential Diagnosis of the Electrocardiogram*)

Dr D. Benazon and the editor of *Anaesthesia* for Fig. 82

Dr G.E. Burch and Henry Kimpton, London for Fig. 8 (from *A Primer of Electrocardiography*)

Dr J.H. Cannard and the editor of *Anesthesiology* for Fig. 72

Dr J. Cox for Fig. 84

Dr C.R. Dundas for Figs. 93 (a) and (c)

Dr J.L. Eiseman and the editor of the *American Journal of Surgery* for Fig. 87

Dr M. Johnstone and the editor of the *British Journal of Anaesthesia* for Figs. 69, 70, 71, 74

Professor C.A. Keele and Professor E. Neil and Oxford Medical Publications for Figs. 5. 7, 13 (from Samson Wright's *Applied Physiology*, 10th ed.)

Dr B.R. Kennedy for Fig. 67

Dr D.M. Krikler and the editor of the *Lancet* for Figs. 1, 2 and 68

Professor S.D. Larks and C.C. Thomas, Springfield, Illinois for Fig. 16 (from *Fetal Electrocardiography*)

Dr B.S. Lipman and Year Book Medical Publishers Inc. Chicago for Figs. 2, 17, 22, 25, 41, 48, 49, 57, 62, 65, 66 (from *Clinical Unipolar Electrocardiography*, 4th edn.)

Dr K. Lupprian, Dr H. Churchill-Davidson and the editor of *The British Medical Journal* for Fig. 60

Dr J.G. Mudd and the editor of the *American Heart Journal* for Fig. 83

Dr C.C. Richards for Fig. 85

Dr J.E.F. Riseman and the Macmillan Company, New York for Figs. 6 (a), (b), (c), 15

Professor L. Schamroth and Blackwell Scientific Publications, Oxford for Figs. 4, 18, 86 (from *An Introduction to Electrocardiography*)

Dr C.F. Scurr and the editor of the *Proceedings of the Royal Society of Medicine* for Fig. 80

Dr D.S. Short for Figs. 47, 63

Dr W.D. Wylie and Lloyd-Luke Ltd, London for Figs. 24, 80 (from *A Practice of Anaesthesia*)

1

INTRODUCTION

Aristotle noted electrical phenomena associated with living tissues, but it is only in the last two centuries that a systematic study of electrophysiology has developed. In 1901 Einthoven was able to measure the electrical activity of the heart and this resulted in the birth of electrocardiography. Although an ECG was taken during surgery as early as 1918 it was not until 1932 that Hill studied the dysrhythmias occurring during chloroform anaesthesia. The application of the ECG as a routine during anaesthesia was introduced by Johnstone in 1948. The use of the ECG has increased to such an extent that all major surgery is done with ECG monitoring.

To interpret the ECG, the anaesthetist needs to know the mechanism producing the electrical activity of the heart which produced the normal ECG pattern. This pattern is modified by disease of the heart and can also suffer transient changes. These occur frequently during anaesthesia and surgery. The anaesthetist has to interpret the clinical ECG preoperatively to decide whether any special measures are indicated in planning the anaesthetic technique. In the theatre, transient changes may occur and these must be interpreted. Very similar problems occur during Intensive Care and the anaesthetist will need to use ECG data in supervising the patient. The development of new anaesthetic techniques involves an assessment of potential risk and the ECG is a valuable tool in this type of research.

ELECTROPHYSIOLOGY

Cells of excitable tissues have a polarized membrane with a negative charge inside and a positive charge outside in the resting state. Most cells need a stimulus, usually electrical, to change the electrical state of the

1

cell. After such a stimulus the voltage across the membrane, called the transmembrane potential, changes in the way shown in figure 1(a). The cycle is divided into five phases. The resting state is known as Phase 4 and the transmembrane potential is about −90 mV. The applied shock reduces this potential and if the reduction is sufficient a rapid reversal of

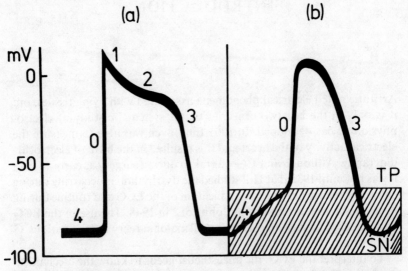

Fig. 1. Transmembrane action potentials. (a) Myocardial cells; (b) cells from the sinoatrial node (TP = threshold potential; SN = supernormal phase).

voltage takes place; the critical potential needed for this to occur is called the threshold potential. The electrical activity of the cycle corresponds to ion movements across the cell membrane.

Phase 0. This is the period of rapid depolarization when sodium ions migrate into the cell. The reversal of potential is called the overshoot. The duration of phase 0 is very brief, usually about 1 ms.

Phase 1. This is the phase of rapid repolarization when calcium ions start to migrate into the cell.

Phase 2. The inflow of calcium ions continues but the potential remains nearly constant and is called the plateau.

Phase 3. During this second period of rapid repolarization potassium ions migrate out of the cell.

Phase 4. This phase has a constant potential and continues at this potential until the cell is stimulated again. During this phase potassium ions migrate inwards and sodium ions outwards until equilibrium is reached.

The entire sequence of potential change from the beginning of depolarization to the end of repolarization forms an action potential. For myocardial cells, the duration of the action potential is much longer than for nerve or muscle fibres. For most of the period of the action potential, the cell will not respond to a further stimulus. Until the transmembrane potential reaches a certain voltage, it is absolutely refractory, and between that voltage and the resting level, a larger stimulus is usually needed, the cell being relatively refractory. In some cells there may be a period before repolarization is complete when the cell is more sensitive to a stimulus; this is called the super-normal phase and is mainly found in cells in the Purkinje fibres.

Whilst the above pattern applies for the great majority of myocardial cells, there are some cells for which in Phase 4 the potential does not remain constant but decreases spontaneously (diastolic depolarization). Eventually the potential rises above the threshold value and depolarization recurs spontaneously. These cells thus have a cycle of depolarization, repolarization, slow change followed by depolarization and the whole cycle repeats. Such cells are called automatic cells. The cycle of a typical automatic cell is shown in figure 1(b). Phase 0 lasts longer and Phases 1 and 2 merge into a more rounded repolarization potential. Automatic cells are potential pacemakers. The cycle length for automatic cells varies and usually increases moving through the conducting system from the SA node to the Purkinje fibres. If an automatic cell is stimulated either during the later part of Phase 3 or Phase 4 it will depolarize at that point and so will have its automaticity overridden by the stimulus.

Changes in the mechanism ions can move across the cell membrane will change the action potential of the cell. Ultimately, the effect of pharmacological agents on the action of the heart must be explained in these terms.

Having examined a mechanism for the electrical behaviour of a single cell it is now necessary to consider the way that the electrical behaviour of the entire heart is constructed from the cooperative behaviour of many cells. This is the electrical anatomy of the heart.

ELECTRICAL ANATOMY

The anatomy of the heart has distinguished many separate features and it is clear that this anatomical description enables the electrical conduction system to be described. The normal heart has a pacemaker in the sinoatrial (SA) node and this must be an automatic cell. This stimulus then passes to the atrioventricular (AV) node along the internodal tracts. The internodal tracts are three bands of tissue; in electrical terms

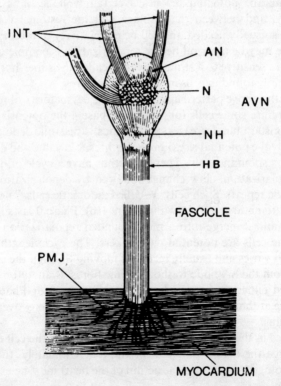

Fig. 2. Diagram to show internodal tracts (ITN), atrioventricular node (AVN) with proximal (AN), central (N) and distal (NH) regions and bundle of His (HB). Terminal fascicles reach the myocardium via complex Purkinje myocardial junctions (PMJ).

this gives three alternative paths for the impulse to get from the SA to the AV node.

The conduction system in the AV node is more complex as the AV node can be split into three zones, AN, N and NH (figure 2). The AN zone receives the impulse and transmits it to the lattice like the N zone. The N zone has a low conduction velocity and this also means that very high atrial rates can be blocked because the subsequent impulse arrives during the refractory period. The N zone connects the AV node with the bundle of His. From the bundle of His the conduction system becomes complex (figure 3). The major path to the right ventricle is the right bundle branch (RBB), and to the left ventricle there are two major paths — the anterior (LAD) and posterior (LPD) divisions of the left bundle branch (LBB). The left bundle branch also includes a centroseptal division. However, a more detailed study shows that a variety of alternative paths exist giving the possibility of conduction when a main route is blocked.

In the ventricles, the RBB and LBB terminate in the Purkinje network

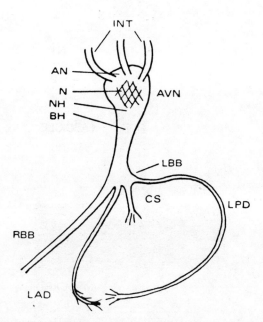

Fig. 3. Diagram to complement figure 2 by showing the left bundle branch (LBB), the centroseptal division (CS), the left posterior division (LPD), the left anterior division (LAD) and the right bundle branch (RBB).

which conveys the impulses to the ventricular muscle. On receiving the impulse, the ventricles contract completing the electrical conduction and producing the mechanical effect. The Purkinje fibres have the highest conduction velocity, thus ensuring that the contraction of the ventricle has a high mechanical efficiency.

The above description is a simplified account of the normal electrical activity of the heart. Not only do other conduction paths exist but there are automatic cells distributed throughout the heart. For more detailed discussion see Krikler and Goodwin (1975).

The great complexity of the electrical system permits a wide variety of abnormal patterns of electrical activity to occur. Abnormal electrical patterns reflect both the failure of the normal conduction path of the heart and mechanisms which nevertheless still cause rhythmical contractions of the ventricles.

2

THE NORMAL ECG

In Chapter 1 the electrophysiology of the heart has been discussed. As the heart is not directly accessible the electric behaviour of the heart is usually deduced from measurements made at the surface of the body. As a first approximation the heart can be considered as an electric dipole, varying cyclically in magnitude and direction, embedded in a poorly conducting homogeneous medium, i.e. the body. Electrical theory shows that such a dipole will produce cyclically fluctuating potentials at all points on the surface of the body. Thus by measuring potentials at different points on the body surface it should be possible to deduce the electric activity of the heart.

Early in this century Einthoven (1903) developed a sufficiently sensitive recording technique to enable him to confirm the existence of electric potentials at the body surface corresponding to the heart's electrical activity. The possibility of measuring electric potentials related to the heart's activity led to the conclusion that these potentials had diagnostic value in the study of heart disease, and to the development of standard methods of recording cardiac activity by using electrodes in standard positions. The interpretation of the patterns obtained developed rather as an art than a science but the cardiologist found that he had a valuable tool. The recording instrument acquired the name of an electrocardiograph and the tracing became known as an electrocardiogram usually shortened to ECG.

This empirical development has led to an almost standard ECG technique. Many research scientists feel that different approaches would yield more accurate data on the state of the heart, but it is difficult to change a convention so firmly established. Of all the suggestions the most persistent is that vectorcardiography would be more satisfactory. Although both the theory and instrumentation of this method have been

7

in existence for many years it is only a very small group of enthusiasts who in fact use it. Alternative axis systems are discussed by Bourdillon (1977). Only scalar electrocardiography will be discussed in this book. An intensive study of ECGs has been made by cardiologists and in this and the next chapter a brief summary of their findings for normal and abnormal hearts will be presented. Fuller details can be found in standard works on electrocardiography, and atlases of typical ECGs found in particular cardiac disorders have been published (Büchner *et al*, 1977; Fleming, 1979). Dubin (1971) has endeavoured to make the rapid interpretation of ECGs simple.

THE ECG LEADS

It is not possible to measure a potential but only the potential difference between two points. Einthoven introduced the use of two electrodes sited at different positions on the body and so measured an ECG between these two points. In order to compare patterns either for the same patient on different occasions or for different patients the lead had to be sited in simple identifiable positions. Not surprisingly the limbs were chosen for the first set of standard positions. The use of the limbs produced the classic standard leads I, II and III.

Standard leads

The right arm, the left arm and the left leg were chosen as electrode sites and are denoted by RA, LA and LF respectively (initially in fact the left foot was used, hence the abbreviation LF). The electrodes were connected in pairs to give the standard leads:

Lead I: LA-RA
Lead II: LF-RA
Lead III: LF-LA

The first of each pair is the positive electrode. A hypothetical line joining the poles of a lead is known as the axis of the lead.

Technically only two of these leads are required as the third is only the difference between the other two and gives no new information. Clinically however, it is convenient to have all three displayed because particular complexes may be very small in a given lead.

Both in practice and theoretically the actual position of the electrode on the arm or leg makes no significant difference to the ECG. The potentials at these electrodes are effectively the potentials at the two shoulders and the top of the thigh. Following Einthoven these positions are idealized to an equilateral triangle centred on the heart (figure 4). For an equilateral triangle the sum of the potentials at the three corners is zero, and in practice the sum of the potentials at the three standard electrodes is effectively zero. This means that a neutral electrode can be obtained by connecting all three together (figure 4). The use of these

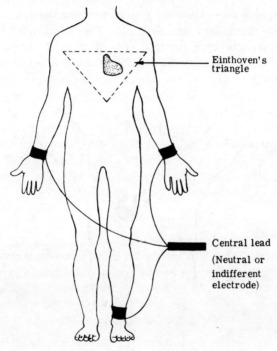

Einthoven's triangle

Central lead

(Neutral or indifferent electrode)

Fig. 4. Einthoven's triangle and the central terminal.

leads showed that for each cycle of the heart there were three main electrical changes: a P wave corresponding to atrial depolarization, a complicated electrical pattern, the QRS complex, corresponding to ventricular depolarization and a T wave corresponding to repolarization of the ventricles. In addition, the T wave is sometimes followed by a U wave whose origin is not clear. The magnitude and direction of the various waves depend on which standard lead is recorded.

Unipolar leads

If a neutral electrode is available then the potential difference between this and any other electrode will give the actual potential of that electrode. Such a measurement is called unipolar compared with the bipolar measurement between two electrodes, each of whose potential varies. The standard leads are bipolar and by using them to form a neutral electrode unipolar leads can be formed with the exploring electrode at any desired location.

Unipolar limb leads. These are formed by using the neutral electrode and one of the standard limb electrodes. They are denoted by VR, VL and VF where the limb electrode is right arm, left arm and left leg respectively. The potentials are usually small and thus difficult to interpret (figure 5).

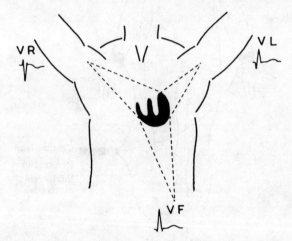

Fig. 5. The right arm lead faces the cavity of the ventricle, the left leg lead faces the inferior surface of the heart; this may be formed by the right or left ventricle or both, depending on the position of the heart. The left arm lead may face the cavity of the ventricles or the outside of the left ventricle, depending on the position of the heart. (Diagram by Dr D.S. Short).

Augmented limb leads. These increase the potential difference compared with the unipolar limb leads by omitting the particular electrode concerned from the neutral electrode. They are known as AVR, AVL and AVF. These are not true unipolar leads.

Precordial leads. The second type of unipolar lead is a precordial lead and utilizes an exploring electrode to record the electrical potentials of the right ventricle, septum and left ventricle. The unipolar chest leads are designated by the single capital letter V, followed by a numeral which represents the location of the electrode on the precordium. Six chest positions are routinely used (V1–6):

V1   4th intercostal space to the right of the sternum
V2   4th intercostal space to the left of the sternum
V3   Midway between the left sternal border and midclavicular line on a line joining positions 2 and 4
V4   5th intercostal space in the midclavicular line
V5   5th intercostal space in the left anterior axillary line
V6   5th intercostal space in the midaxillary line

The position of the chest leads are illustrated in figures 6(a), (b) and (c).

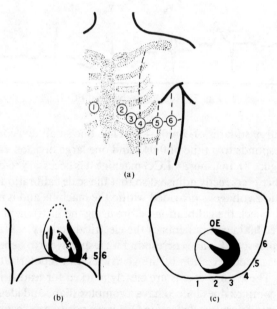

Fig. 6. The normal ECG. (a) Position of the exploring electrodes on the precordium. (b) The cardiac structures visualized by the precordial exploring electrodes. (c) The cardiac structure visualized by both the precordial electrodes and the oesophageal electrode (OE).

APPEARANCE OF THE NORMAL ECG

The cardiologist normally takes a twelve-lead ECG on a patient. The leads are: the standard leads I, II and III, the augmented limb leads AVR, AVL and AVF and the precordial leads V1–6. A typical set of tracings is shown in figure 7. Conventionally, the size of ECG tracings has been standardized for ease of interpretation. The potential difference is shown as the vertical deflection with a scale of 10 mm corresponding to 1 mV and the horizontal scale represents the time to a scale of 25 mm to 1 s. The recording paper is graduated in small squares of 1-mm

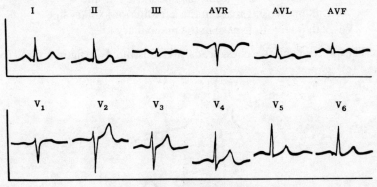

Fig. 7. Normal twelve-lead ECG.

side and large squares of 5-mm side. Thus one small division horizontally corresponds to a time of 0·04 s and one large division vertically to 0·5 mV (figure 8). In using an ECG machine it is necessary to ensure that the amplifier is correctly adjusted so that the scale calibration is correct. A calibration voltage is provided within the machine and it is standard practice to check the calibration before using the instrument.

The three main components of the electrical activity are the P wave, QRS complex and T wave corresponding respectively to depolarization of the atria, depolarization of the ventricles and repolarization of the ventricles. These three events are clearly marked for lead II in figure 9. The QRS complex does indeed have a complex shape and ideally has the form of a small negative deflection Q, a large positive deflection R and a small negative deflection S. Following the T wave, the diagram shows a small positive wave known as the U wave. The U wave is frequently absent and its origin is obscure.

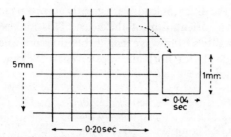

Fig. 8. Time markings and voltage lines of the electrocardiogram.

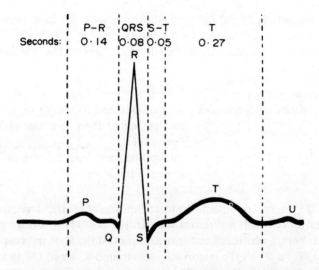

Fig. 9. Normal limb lead tracing illustrating the intervals.

The diagram indicates the duration of the significant phases of the ECG. The shape of the QRS complex is such that it is often difficult to measure the time of commencement of the Q and S waves; hence the interval between the onset of the P wave and that of the QRS complex is often measured as PR rather than PQ.

The examination of ECGs show that no two are absolutely alike and so the cardiologist needs considerable experience to know when to regard a tracing as abnormal. Experience has shown that for most components normal ranges can be specified. The height of the ECG components in the different leads vary greatly according to the mechanical and electrical orientation of the heart. This makes it difficult to deduce abnormalities from wave heights but does not affect the various intervals. Standards for normality are given with some precision for intervals as follows:

Duration of P wave	up to 110 ms
PR interval	100–200 ms
Width of QRS complex	50–100 ms
ST interval	50 ms
QT interval	400 ms
Duration of T wave	270 ms

The magnitude of the components varies with the lead; precordial leads usually have a higher voltage and unipolar limb leads a lower voltage than the standard leads. Standards of normality for the standard leads are:

Height of P wave	2·5 mm (0·25 mV)
Height of QRS complex	at least 5·0 mm (0·5 mV) in any lead and no higher than 15·0 mm (1·5 mV) in any lead
Height of T wave	this should be at least 2·0 mm (0·2 mV) in one of the leads

The QT interval represents the total duration of ventricular activation and recovery time. It is often standardized as the QTc to a heart rate of 60 beats per min by dividing the square root of the R–R interval 'c' i.e. $QTc = QT\sqrt{c}$. The QTc is normally less than 0·42 s and QT is usually less than half the R–R interval except at extremes of rate.

The end of the T wave is best defined in lead AVL where the U wave is usually isoelectric.

Returning to figure 7 it will be seen that all twelve leads have different characteristics. One of the standard leads, usually lead III, will have low voltage; generally lead II has a large voltage and is commonly used for ECG monitoring. The augmented limb leads are approximately unipolar and so estimate the electric potential in three directions from the heart. The precordial leads are unipolar leads and so measure the electric potential at a number of points close to the heart itself. Hence the big difference seen in the ECG should be related to the momentary direction of the dipole equivalent to the heart. If an electric vector is directed towards an electrode a positive potential is produced, if away from it a negative potential and if perpendicular to it no potential. In these leads it is the shape of the QRS complex which varies most strikingly. This is due to the fact that the path of depolarization through the ventricles is a complex one, first going through the septum and then the two ventricles (figure 10). Figures 11 and 12 show the potential difference produced by the passage of a depolarization pulse through the normal ventricles at an

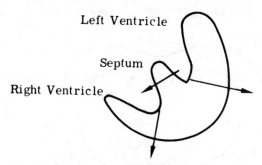

Fig. 10. Mechanism of ventricular depolarization.

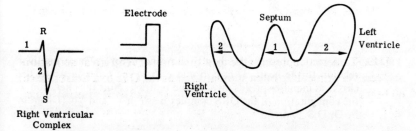

Fig. 11. The right ventricular complex. (In the normal heart the larger left ventricular forces counteract and in effect nullify the smaller forces of the right ventricle so that septal depolarization (1) and left ventricular depolarization (2) need only be considered.)

electrode placed on opposite sides of the ventricles. Figure 13 shows the relation between precordial electrodes and a normally orientated ventricle. The change in pattern observed as the electrode overlies the septum (V_3 in figure 7) is known as the transitional zone.

By convention any negative wave following an R wave is the S wave. If more than one R or S wave occurs the further waves are designated R[1] or

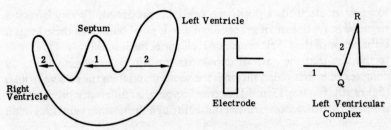

Fig. 12. The left ventricular complex.

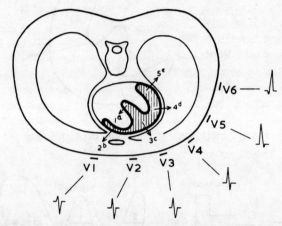

Fig. 13. Cross-section through the chest to show the precordial leads and their relation to the heart; a, b, c, d and e show the order in which the electrical impulse spreads through the ventricle. Note the alteration in the configuration of the QRS complex between V1 and V6. (Diagram by Dr D.S. Short.)

r^1 or S^1 or s^1 depending on their relative size. These can usually be observed in bundle branch block (figures 48 and 49).

A QRS in the form of a single negative wave is known as a QS complex.

The base line of the ECG, i.e. the PR and TP intervals, is known as the isoelectric line.

THE ELECTRIC AXIS

As the electrical activity of the heart is a vector quantity, the magnitude of the signal in any lead depends on the direction of the electric vector as well as its magnitude. Thus if only one standard lead is used a small QRS complex does not necessarily mean that the electrical activity of the ventricle is weak; it may in fact be strong but the electric vector may be almost perpendicular to the direction of this lead. Considerations like this are the justification for suggesting that vectorcardiography would be a great improvement on the usual ECG. However, it is possible to estimate the direction of the electric axis by using the standard leads. The use of computers makes it possible to calculate the instantaneous magnitude and direction of the component of the electric vector in the vertical plane from two standard leads. Mean values of this component can be calculated for the QRS complex and the T wave in relatively simple ways (Rollason and Hough 1957a).

Clinically it is relatively easy to estimate the mean axis of the QRS complex by inspecting the standard and augmented limb leads. From the Einthoven triangle (figure 4) the direction of the three standard leads is along the three sides of a equilateral triangle; a little thought shows that the augmented limb leads will have directions at right angles to the standard leads. Figure 14 shows the direction of these six leads; the

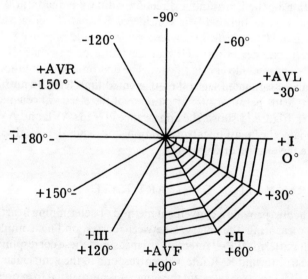

Fig. 14. The hexaxial reference system. Hatched area indicates the normal range of the electric axis. The convention of labelling this system as positive and negative units should not be confused with the positive and negative poles of the lead axes.

electric axis is considered to be in its normal position in the direction of lead I and this is taken as the zero of axis deviation. Clockwise rotations are considered to be positive and anticlockwise negative. The deflection in a lead can be either positive or negative and figure 14 shows the twelve directions of the electric vector if it is parallel to one of the leads. This system of six axes is called a hexaxial reference system, and if the standard leads are used alone the reference system is a triaxial one.

If a lead is accurately perpendicular to the electric vector there will be no signal in that lead. Inspection of the standard and augmented leads will show which lead has the smallest QRS complex; the lead perpendicular to this (figure 14) should have the largest QRS magnitude and will be approximately in the direction of the electric axis. The sign of the QRS complex removes the uncertainty as to direction and so the mean electric axis is located within $\pm 15°$. The magnitude and sign of the QRS complex in the lead where it is smallest will enable a precise estimate to be made of the electric axis if this is desired. Without any measurement of QRS voltages, by inspection, the mean electric axis can be located within $\pm 5°$.

The position of the electric axis is not simply related to the anatomical orientation of the heart and a direction within the quadrant $0°$ to $90°$ (hatched area in figure 14) is considered normal. Positive values of greater than $90°$ are called right axis deviation and negative values are called left axis deviation. Left axis deviation of less than $30°$ is not normally considered very significant. The anatomical orientation of the heart can be estimated from the augmented limb leads (figure 7). The standard leads permit a similar estimate of the electrical orientation of the heart. Figure 15 shows the appearance of leads AVL and AVF used to estimate the anatomical orientation and leads I and III used to estimate the electric orientation.

DETERMINATION OF HEART RATE

ECG tracings provide a convenient method of determining heart rate by simply measuring the interval between corresponding complexes in adjacent patterns. If P–P intervals are measured these correspond to the atrial heart rate and R–R intervals correspond to the ventricular rate; in a stable ECG the two rates are the same. It is more usual to express heart rate, B, as beats per minute rather than in terms of the duration, T, of one beat in seconds. The ECG measurement of T is easily converted into the standard form by the formula:

$$B=\frac{60}{T}$$

A quick estimate of the rate can also be obtained by dividing the number of 0·20 s intervals between complexes into 300.

Some ECG paper is marked at 3·0 s intervals (15 large squares) and the rate is readily obtained by multiplying the number of complexes between these intervals by twenty.

Many ECG monitors incorporate a rate meter which electrically measures the heart rate.

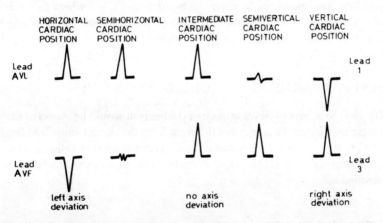

Fig. 15. The five patterns of augmented limb leads which indicate the cardiac position compared with the three patterns in the standard leads indicating axis deviation (Chapter 3).

MONITORING THE ECG

The cardiologist uses a twelve-lead ECG as a matter of routine. It is rarely possible to continuously record all twelve leads when, as in anaesthesia, it is desired to monitor the ECG over a period of time. Most monitor displays will only present one or two leads and in addition it is not convenient to use so many electrodes on the patient. This means it is necessary to decide which leads will give the most satisfactory representation of the ECG in these circumstances. Reference to figure 7 shows that the normal ECG has a good pattern in lead II and this is probably the most commonly used monitoring lead. One advantage is that the standard lead electrodes are fairly remote from the heart and are unlikely to interfere with other apparatus and procedures. There have been suggestions that lead II may produce spurious ST segment data because the repolarization of the atrium (Ta wave) takes place during this period and has its maximum effect in lead II. During surgery, the lead used must depend on the surgical requirements and so it is not possible to standardize on a single lead. During anaesthesia dysrhythmias are probably more important than the magnitude of the components. It is helpful to be able to use past experience (of others and of oneself) in the interpretation of a particular pattern. This suggests that lead II should be used when possible, although others prefer the bipolar lead CM5 where the reference electrode is situated over the manubrium sterni and the exploring electrode in the precordial lead V5 position.

ECG PATTERNS IN THE CHILD AND FETUS

During the period of development of the heart, it would be expected that the pattern would be somewhat different from that in the adult. The fetal ECG is difficult to record because the ECG of the mother will also occur in the tracing (figure 16). Rapid progress is being made in fetal electrocardiography.

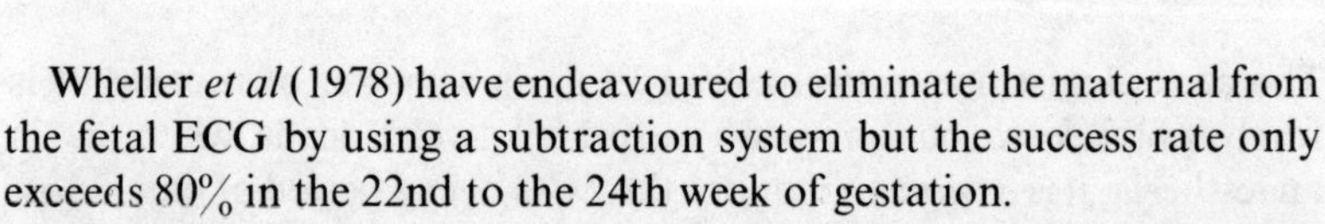

Fig. 16. Maternal complexes (M) and fetal complexes (F) in the ECG.

Wheller *et al* (1978) have endeavoured to eliminate the maternal from the fetal ECG by using a subtraction system but the success rate only exceeds 80% in the 22nd to the 24th week of gestation.

The ECG of the newborn infant is very similar to the fetal ECG and gradually changes into the adult pattern. Figure 17 gives the ECG pattern for a normal child and should be compared with figure 7 (normal adult ECG).

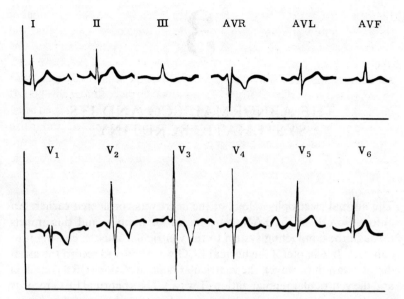

Fig. 17. Normal ECG in boy aged 2. Note the inverted T waves in V1, V2, and V3 which are normal at this age.

3

THE ABNORMAL ECG AND ITS
SYSTEMATIC SCRUTINY

The normal electrophysiology of the heart was considered earlier. An automatic cell in the SA node initiates an impulse and this travels through the conducting system to the ventricular muscle, causing it to contract. In Chapter 2 the normal ECG was shown to record the atrial depolarization (P wave), the ventricular depolarization (QRS complex) and the ventricular repolarization (T wave). The abnormal ECG records the changes in magnitude, duration and interval between these components. To interpret the ECG these changes must be related to changes in the electrical activity of the heart. The two main types of change are alteration in the site of the automatic cell acting as pacemaker and changes in the conduction. Changes in the site of the pacemaker will cause dysrhythmias. The effect of changes in the conduction are more complex; they may affect the magnitude of the components, the interval between them and also cause dysrhythmias.

Although it is increasingly possible to explain the appearance of the ECG in terms of electrophysiology, cardiologists over many years have developed an empirical interpretation of the ECG. This chapter is mainly concerned with this empirical approach but some reference will be made to theory where appropriate. The chapter concludes with a method for the systematic scrutiny of the twelve-lead ECG.

Of the twelve-lead ECG, the P wave is usually most prominent in leads II and V1. If it is difficult to observe the P wave some additional leads may be used. Two bipolar leads are used; S5 and MCL1. The S5 lead uses the lead I terminals with one electrode sited over the right fifth interspace adjacent to the sternum instead of the left arm and the other electrode over the manubrium instead of the right arm. The MCL1 lead has the positive electrode at the V1 position and the negative electrode on the left shoulder just under the outer end of the clavicle. The unipolar lead has the electrode in the oesophagus. It is usually positioned to produce the maximum amplitude of P wave.

ALTERATIONS IN THE P WAVE

The P wave is tall and sharp, the height ranging from 2 to 5 mm (0·2 to 0·5 mV) in right atrial hypertrophy, e.g. in pulmonary stenosis and is referred to as P pulmonale.

It is usually bifid and conspicuously widened—the duration being in the region of 0·12 s (120 ms)—in left atrial hypertrophy, e.g. in mitral stenosis, and is referred to as P mitrale (figure 18).

When the P wave is enlarged in association with the right ventricular hypertrophy due to congenital heart disease it is known as P congenitale. It is widened and the voltage is low in hypertensive and aortic valve disease. In lead I it is inverted in dextrocardia. This is illustrated in figure 19.

Lead II **Lead V₁**

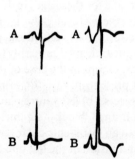

Fig. 18. ECG tracings show the features of left and right atrial enlargement. A = left atrial enlargement, B = right atrial enlargement.

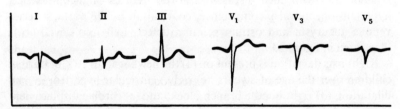

Fig. 19. Congenital dextrocardia. Lead I is the mirror image of normal lead I; leads II and III are reversed and leads V3 and V5 resemble the right precordial leads.

The configuration of the P wave frequently changes in height and direction when the pacemaker shifts from the sinus node to various portions of the atrium, and the PR interval varies (figure 39). This phenomenon is called wandering pacemaker and will be referred to again under ectopic rhythm.

It may be absent in sino-atrial block, atrial fibrillation, hyperkalaemia and AV nodal rhythm.

ALTERATIONS MAINLY AFFECTING THE QRS COMPLEX

AXIS DEVIATION

The direction of the mean normal electrical axis varies considerably with the age of the subject. In the infant under 6 months of age, the axis is greatly to the right (+ 130°). Between the ages of 1 and 5 years, the axis moves to the left, the average for these ages inclusive being about + 52°. The axis then returns to the right at puberty, the average axis being about + 67°. It again returns to the left in the adult, averaging about + 58°. These changes in position are due mainly to the changing position of the heart in the thorax, except in the case of the infant.

Left axis deviation is present in: (a) 10% of normal people who are usually hypersthenic subjects; (b) left ventricular hypertrophy and dilatation, (c) left bundle branch block—significant left axis deviation (− 30° to − 120°) is due to an intraventricular conduction defect involving the anterior-superior division of the left bundle branch (left anterior hemiblock); and (d) cardiac displacement to the left, e.g. due to scoliosis, elevation of the diaphragm as a result of pregnancy, obesity or ascites. It is associated with such diseases as aortic stenosis or incompetence, hypertension, mitral incompetence, coarctation of the aorta, arterio-venous aneurysm and ostium primum defect. Left axis deviation is illustrated in figure 20.

Right axis deviation is present in: (a) the newborn; (b) 10% of normal children over the age of 8 years; (c) right ventricular hypertrophy and dilatation; (d) right bundle branch block; and (e) cardiac displacement to the right. It is associated with such diseases as emphysema, mitral and pulmonary stenosis and ostium secundum defects. Right axis deviation is illustrated in figure 21.

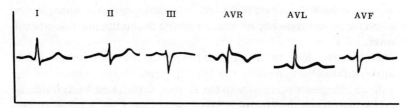

Fig. 20. Left axis deviation (leads I and III). Horizontal heart (leads AVL and AVF).

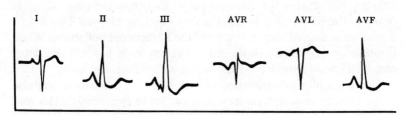

Fig. 21. Right axis deviation (leads I and III). Vertical heart (leads AVL and AVF).

VOLTAGE CHANGES

An excessively high or low voltage of the QRS complex may be due to a standardization error and this should be checked. On the other hand it may be related to the thickness of the chest wall and to disease.

High voltage may be seen in patients with (a) a thin chest wall, (b) ventricular hypertrophy, and (c) hyperthyroidism.

Low voltage may be seen in patients with (a) a thick chest wall, (b) a pericardial effusion, anasarca, myocarditis or myopathy, (c) myxoedema, (d) carbon monoxide poisoning and (e) emphysema.

LEFT VENTRICULAR HYPERTROPHY

This is classically seen in patients with hypertension and is associated with left axis deviation. The diagnostic electrocardiographic signs are:

1. The R wave is likely to exceed 15 mm (1·5 mV) in one of the standard leads because of the generation of excess voltage.

2. The tall R wave is followed by an inverted T wave. When the myocardium is severely hypertrophied or 'strained' it has been conjectured that repolarization is so retarded in its progress through the

affected myocardium that other areas repolarize earlier. Consequently, a reverse progression occurs which imparts to the tracing a negative T wave.

3. There is a delay in the onset of the downstroke of the R wave (the intrinsicoid deflection) over the left ventricular leads. Almost all the voltage changes concerned with the R wave in the chest leads normally take place during the upstroke. The downstroke of the R merely represents the time it takes for the detector to return to zero with no electric current flowing. In heart strain, delay in depolarization results in voltage changes even during the downstroke, so that from the peak of the R down to the base line, a longer than normal time elapses. This downstroke, as indicated above, is termed the intrinsicoid deflection. When the intrinsicoid deflection is slurred in the chest leads, however, the delay characteristic of hypertrophy is obvious without measurement.

The ventricular activation time (VAT) is the time taken for an impulse to traverse the myocardium from endocardial to epicardial surface and is reflected in the measurement of the time interval from the beginning of the Q to the peak of the R and is prolonged when the onset of the intrinsicoid deflection is delayed.

4. In addition to the QRS and T wave changes the ST segment is frequently below the isoelectric line.

With left ventricular strain, high R and negative ST and T occur in left ventricular positions i.e, V5 and V6, and this is illustrated in figure 22 and may be seen in hypertensive heart disease and aortic stenosis.

RIGHT VENTRICULAR HYPERTROPHY

This is usually associated with right axis deviation and the diagnostic electrocardiographic signs are:

1. Increased voltage of the R wave over the right ventricular leads and the S waves over the left precordial leads are greater than normal.

2. A QR pattern may be present in lead AVR. This may be due to marked clockwise rotation, so that the left ventricle faces AVR, or the possibility that, in right ventricular hypertrophy, lead AVR faces a portion of the right ventricle and consequently faces the depolarization wave more directly. The diagnosis of right ventricular hypertrophy, therefore, may be made when the QRS complex of AVR is more positive than negative, and about 50% of all patients with an R as high as 4 mm (0·4 mV) have right ventricular strain, no matter how negative the Q or S

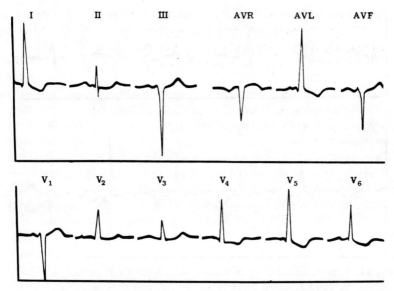

Fig. 22. Left ventricular hypertrophy ('strain pattern').

may be. Moreover, a positive T in AVR is abnormal and may indicate right strain.

3. Delayed onset of the intrinsicoid deflection over the right ventricular leads.

4. Depression of the ST segment and inversion of the T wave over the right ventricular positions i.e. V1 and V2, but here a normal negative T wave must be differentiated.

Right ventricular hypertrophy with strain is illustrated in figure 23 and may be seen in pulmonary embolism and chronic pulmonary disease.

Biventricular hypertrophy may occur, e.g. in ventricular septal defect, resulting in large amplitude diphasic QRS complexes in many leads. This is known as the Katz Wachtel phenomenon.

BUNDLE BRANCH BLOCK

This condition, which may be permanent, intermittent or transient, is due to a block in one of the branches of the bundle of His. When the QRS complex is 0·12 s (120 ms) or more, complete bundle branch block is present. If between 0·10 and 0·12 s (100 ms and 120 ms) incomplete

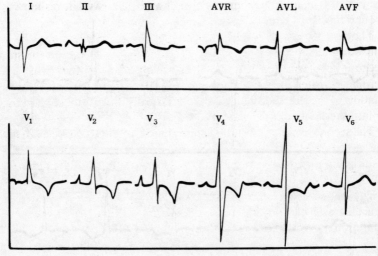

Fig. 23. Right ventricular hypertrophy ('strain pattern'). P. pulmonale in leads V2 and V3.

bundle branch block may be said to exist. Bundle branch block is primarily an electrocardiographic diagnosis and may occur in clinically normal hearts.

Bundle branch block is divided into right and left block. In typical block the T wave is opposite to the main part of the QRS complex, but in atypical block the converse holds. Bundle branch block will be discussed further under disorders of cardiac rhythm.

ELECTRICAL ALTERNANS

This is an alteration of high and low QRS complexes. It is not significant unless the heart rate is slow. This abnormality does not produce any disturbances.

ALTERATIONS MAINLY AFFECTING THE ST SEGMENT AND T WAVE

MYOCARDIAL INFARCTION

This probably results in three physiologically abnormal zones. The centre is the zone of necrosis (electrically inert), the surrounding area is the zone of injury wherein either healing or necrosis will result, and around this is the zone of ischaemia.

The necrotic centre effects the tracing in two major ways: (a) The R will be small or absent when the electrode subtends necrotic tissue, because depolarization is minimal or absent; and (b) there will be a permanent, often wide, Q wave, because the dead tissue presents an open window to the electrode which is now electrically directly on the septum, or into the cavity of the heart.

The second, or zone of injury, causes the ST interval to be elevated if the electrode is directly over the area, or depressed if more remote resulting in a depressed or elevated base line respectively (Schamroth 1976).

The classical 'current of injury' (the Pardee curve) is illustrated in figure 24 and it is on these raised ST segments that the diagnosis of infarction must be based.

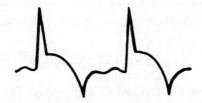

Fig. 24. The Pardee curve.

The third or ischaemic zone causes inversion of the T wave.

Thus there are four changes: small or absent R; deep Q; positive or negative ST; and inverted T.

A full thickness acute infarction of the anterior wall presents all these changes in the precordial leads and is shown in figure 25.

Distinct alterations do not occur in so-called posterior infarction because the active electrode is too remote, but depressed ST segments should make one investigate the posterior infarction in the other leads, particularly leads II and III, and AVF. It should be suspected when there is a deep Q wave and an inverted T wave in these leads.

True posterior infarction, however, has three characteristics:

1. Tall R waves in V1 and V2.
2. Tall symmetrical T waves in V1 and V2.

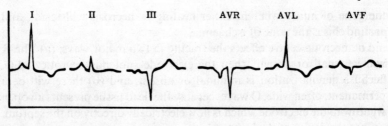

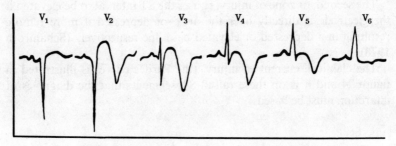

Fig. 25. Diffuse anterior myocardial infarction.

3. Depressed concave-upward ST segments in V1 and V2. The right
   ventricle is very rarely involved.

Very low or absent R, elevated ST and depressed T over positions V5
and V6 indicate lateral infarction; over position V2 or V3, or possibly
V1 also, septal infarction; and over position AVL high anterolateral
infarction.

In all infarctions, the ST usually returns to the isoelectric base line in a
week or two, but the other changes remain for months or years.

In the standard leads, elevations of ST occur rapidly after anterior
infarction in lead I. As the infarction becomes older, the ST descends
towards the base line, but it carries the negative T with it in a characteristic equilimb curve likened to a bird in flight, the final part of the QRS
complex going downwards into the initial segment of the negative T with
a convexity directed upwards. A Q wave in lead I occurs in anterior
infarction, but the R is not much affected. Thus a Q and a negative T in
lead I, with an isoelectric ST indicates an older infarction.

Many infarcts do not show characteristic ECG changes; this is particularly true of lateral infarcts in patients with hypertension. Moreover
in the case of minor or intramural infarctions the ECG may be normal.

In the interpretation of ST elevations or depressions the ST segment is compared with the TP interval following rather than with the PR portion of the base line preceding it. That part of the tracing between the end of the T wave and the beginning of the next P wave is considered the isoelectric level and forms the base line for determining displacement of the ST segment.

Elective surgery should not be undertaken for at least 3 months after a myocardial infarction (Fraser *et al* 1967).

PERICARDITIS

The ECG pattern of pericarditis which causes injury to the subepicardial surface of the heart is best observed in the precordial leads and is characterized by widespread elevation of the ST segments, which maintain their normal upward concavity and the absence of abnormal Q waves. These do not appear since the injury to the heart muscle is superficial. Inverted symmetrical T waves develop after the ST segment returns to the base line. Low voltage of the QRS complexes in all leads may also be observed and is due to the fact that the electric currents in the heart are short-circuited through the pericardial fluid and thickened pericardium.

Figure 26 illustrates the characteristic precordial lead pattern in acute diffuse pericarditis.

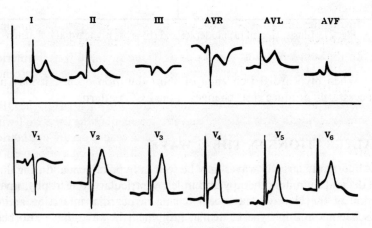

Fig. 26. Acute pericarditis pattern.

MYOCARDIAL ISCHAEMIA

Coronary insufficiency first shows itself in changes in the ST segment and T wave but if persistent also affects the QRS complex. The classical changes are ST depression and T wave flattening or inversion in leads facing the surface of the heart, whereas in leads facing the cavities (usually AVR) there will be a current of injury with raised ST segments. The T wave has a symmetrical limb and a sharp pointed vertex. The change in the QRS complex is likely to be left bundle branch block with significant left axis deviation.

A tendency to myocardial ischaemia will be made evident by taking an ECG after exercise (Kilpatrick 1978).

Myocardial ischaemia is illustrated in figure 27.

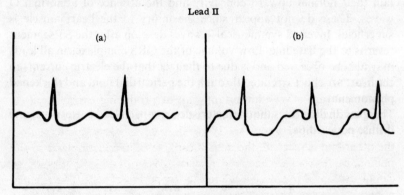

Fig. 27. Illustration of (a) moderate and (b) gross myocardial ischaemia.

When myocardial ischaemia of short duration occurs, it may not necessarily produce clear changes in the ECG pattern.

ALTERATIONS IN THE U WAVE

Abnormally large U waves may be seen in hypokalaemia, during digitalis and quinidine therapy and in left ventricular hypertrophy; inversion of the U wave may occur during myocardial infarction and/or ischaemia and in hyperkalaemia. Prominent U waves have also been associated with hyperventilation (Rollason and Parkes 1957).

DISORDERS OF RHYTHM

Normal sinus rhythm is initiated by a pacemaker in the SA node which sends an impulse through the cardiac system causing the atrium to contract and produce a P wave and later the ventricles contract causing the QRS complex; subsequently the ventricles repolarize to produce a T wave and then the heart is quiescent until the pacemaker fires again. This normal rhythm can be altered in three ways:

1. The cycle length of the pacemaker may increase or decrease or other automatic cells may institute impulses, i.e. disturbances of impulse formation.
2. The speed of conduction in various parts of the path may change or conduction may cease altogether and a block occurs, i.e. disturbances of conduction.
3. A subtle combination of (1) and (2).

Any or all of these events may happen and the result will be a dysrhythmia. At one time, it was thought that the picture could be described in such simple terms but modern work has shown that re-entry phenomena are a very important way of producing extra impulses. These involve the possibility of at least two paths between two points in the heart. An impulse finds one end of the path blocked but by the time the other end is reached, the path is capable of conducting and so the impulse passes back to the initial point of division. This kind of blockage can be explained in terms of the refractory period of cells. The re-entry impulse can act as an impulse which will eventually cause the ventricles to contract.

Any impulse which does not originate at the sino-atrial node is called an ectopic beat. It will travel both to the atrium to cause a P wave and to the ventricle to cause a QRS complex (assuming neither path is blocked). For ectopic beats, the P wave may, of course, appear before, during, or after the QRS complex. It is usual to try and define ectopic beats in terms of the point at which they originate.

At the present time dysrhythmias are the subject of intense reassessment. New names are being given to distinctive ECG patterns in the hope of being a more correct description of what is actually happening. However, there seem to be different theoretical ways of describing the same pattern and the experimental evidence is not adequate to distinguish one theory from another. The use of various forms of intracar-

diac electrogram are gradually enabling the mechanisms to be eluci-
dated but there is still much research to be done. There seems to be little
chance of using intracardiac ECGs as a routine procedure in surgery and
so, for some time yet, it will be necessary for the anaesthetist to continue
to interpret conventional ECGs.

In these circumstances, a fairly conservative description will be given
of dysrhythmias. For a more modern discussion recent works such as
Krikler and Goodwin (1975), Schlant and Hurst (1976) and Hampton
(1977) should be consulted.

Dysrhythmias will be classified into those which are basically modifi-
cations of normal sinus rhythm (physiological) and those involving
ectopic beats or regular rhythms of a non-sinus origin (pathological).

PHYSIOLOGICAL DYSRHYTHMIAS

SINUS DYSRHYTHMIA

This is usually associated with two phases of respiration: during inspiration there is a quickening of impulse formation in the SA node, while
during expiration there is a slowing due to the vagal effect.

Sinus dysrhythmia is most frequently seen in children and young
adults and is usually abolished by atropine and general anaesthesia, but
it may reappear during controlled ventilation. This dysrhythmia is
illustrated in figure 28.

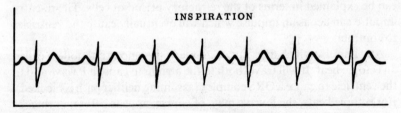

INSPIRATION

Fig. 28. Sinus dysrhythmia.

SINUS TACHYCARDIA

This is associated with an increase in the rate of discharge of impulses
from the SA node in the region of 100 to 160 beats per min in the adult,
and is related to emotional disturbances or exercise. It may also be

associated with diseases such as anaemia, haemorrhage or hyperthyroidism and may occur in the ultra light planes of anaesthesia in the presence of painful stimuli. The TP interval is usually demolished and it becomes necessary to use the PR or the PQ intervals for the isoelectric line.

SINUS BRADYCARDIA

In this condition the SA node discharges at a much slower rate, in the region of 40 to 60 beats per min, and is characteristically seen in the highly trained athlete. Sinus bradycardia may also occur in disease such as myxoedema, obstructive jaundice, raised intracranial pressure and digitalis overdosage.

PATHOLOGICAL DYSRHYTHMIAS

These are classified in Table 1 and are discussed below.

Table 1

Ectopic rhythm		
Extrasystoles	Atrial	
	Nodal	
	Ventricular	
Paroxysmal tachycardia	Atrial	Tachycardia
		Flutter
		Fibrillation
	Nodal	
	Ventricular	Tachycardia
		Flutter
		Fibrillation
Escape rhythm		

Heart block	
Sinoatrial	
Atrioventricular	1st degree
	2nd degree
	3rd degree
Bundle branch block	
Phasic aberrant ventricular	
conduction	

ECTOPIC RHYTHM

Extrasystoles

Atrial.   If the atrium is stimulated during diastole after its refractory period is past, it responds with a premature contraction. An impulse is transmitted to the ventricles which contract too. The P wave is usually abnormal in configuration (e.g. inverted or isoelectric) and the PR interval shortens, but the succeeding ventricular complex is usually normal. The next atrial impulse arising in the SA node appears after a pause equal to the normal diastolic period or a little in excess of it. An atrial extrasystole is illustrated in figure 29. When the atrial beat is so

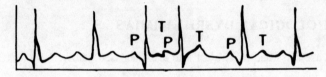

Fig. 29. Atrial extrasystole.

premature that the ventricles are in a refractory state, they fail to respond. Atrial extrasystoles are common during cardiac surgery and appear to have no special significance.

Nodal.   As the ectopic focus is in the AV node both the atria and the ventricles receive conduction impulses originating in the AV node. This means that the P wave will not necessarily occur before the QRS complex; so the P wave may be before or after, or coincide with the QRS complex. The beat occurs prematurely and is followed by a compensatory pause. These are relatively uncommon and of little clinical significance.

Ventricular.   If the ventricle is stimulated during diastole after its refractory period has passed, it also responds with a premature contraction. The ventricular complex is abnormal and is not preceded by a P wave. The next P wave is usually buried within this ventricular complex. The excitation process which arises in the new focus spreads rapidly over the surface of the ventricular muscle in all directions; it also penetrates the ventricular wall to reach the endocardium and so invades the

Purkinje tissue which transmits the excitation process rapidly over its own side of the heart. The same change occurs later in the other ventricle. As the time taken for the excitation process to affect the whole of both ventricles is prolonged, the QRS will exceed 0·12 s in duration; as the pattern of invasion is abnormal, the deflections of the QRS will be abnormal in appearance. The pattern of repolarization is also altered with consequent changes in the ST segment and the T wave. There is no isoelectric portion of the ST segment and the T wave takes off from a level above or below the isoelectric line and usually has a direction opposite to that of the main deflection of the QRS complex. A ventricular extrasystole is illustrated in figure 30. When the ectopic focus originates in the right ventricle, the QRS deflection resembles a left bundle

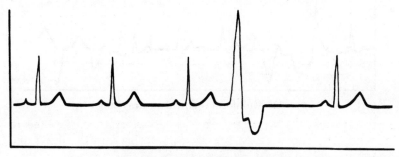

Fig. 30. Ventricular extrasystole.

branch block pattern as seen in the right precordial leads and, when it originates in the left ventricle, the QRS resembles right bundle branch block pattern as seen in the right precordial leads. Ventricular extrasystoles tend to follow long R–R intervals and this is known as the 'Rule of Bigeminy'. The compensatory pause of the extrasystole provides another long R–R interval which tends to produce a further extrasystole so that the process may be self-perpetuating as in bigeminal rhythm (figure 31). Bigeminal rhythm may also be caused by alternate atrial or nodal extrasystoles or by a 3:2 AV block. If ventricular extrasystoles become frequent they interfere with the efficiency of the circulation as the output produced by a premature beat is less than normal because the ventricle has not had time to fill. Multifocal ventricular extrasystoles (figure 32) are usually ominous and may be followed by ventricular fibrillation (figure 33). This may be coarse or fine.

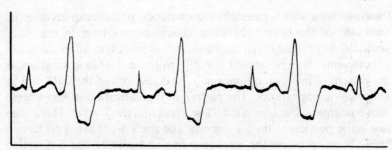

Fig. 31. Pulsus bigeminus.

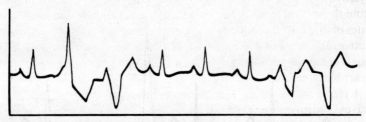

Fig. 32. Multifocal ventricular extrasystoles.

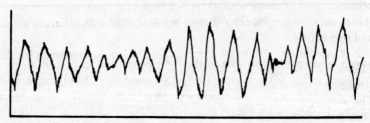

Fig. 33. Ventricular fibrillation (coarse).

Paroxysmal tachycardia

This term is applied to attacks of rapid heart action where ventricular contraction responds to regular impulses arising in a focus removed from the SA node. The rate may be as slow as 100 per min or as rapid as 210, or even faster in infants. Three forms of paroxysmal tachycardia are recognized according to whether the ectopic focus of stimulus formation

is situated in the atrium, AV node or ventricles. The essential characteristics of all types of tachycardia are as follows:

1. They begin suddenly.
2. The first beat is a premature one.
3. The beats are absolutely regular.
4. They terminate suddenly.
5. Carotid sinus pressure, pressure on the eyeball or the administration of a vasopressor, may reduce the rate or stop the paroxysm
   completely.

Atrial. As far as the atrial dysrhythmias are concerned the type of
dysrhythmia produced depends on the rate of discharge of impulses
from the ectopic focus. If the rate is slow, atrial extrasystoles result, but
rates of 100 to 250 produce atrial tachycardia, rates of 260 to 340 atrial
flutter, and rates of 400 to 600 atrial fibrillation. As the AV node can
rarely transmit impulses faster than 210 to 220 per min physiological
heart block results.

   1. *Atrial tachycardia.*   Here there is a rapid succession of abnormal P
waves. The inversion or other deformities of the P wave are explained by
the fact that the impulse causing the contraction does not originate in the
SA node. The change in the P wave may not be noticed until a very close
comparison of the ECG tracing during the attack is made with one taken
before or after. Paroxysmal atrial tachycardia is illustrated in figure 34.
It may occur in pregnancy and may be associated with tobacco, alcohol
and overeating.

   2. *Atrial flutter.*   Here the P waves are absolutely regular in rhythm.
They are characterized by a rapid upstroke and a more gradual downstroke, and by the absence of any iso-electric interval between the waves.
The waves occur in rapid succession usually 260 to 340 per minute but
occasionally as much as 400 per minute. The ratio between atrial and
ventricular complexes is commonly 2:1 as a physiological heart block

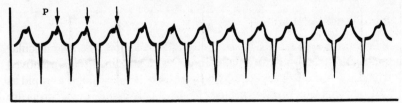

Fig. 34. Paroxysmal atrial tachycardia.

occurs; but the ventricle may respond less frequently so that a 4:1 response is not unusual. When the ratio is 1:1 the tracing is difficult to distinguish from one of paroxysmal atrial tachycardia but in the latter condition the rate is usually less than 210. Figure 35 illustrates a case of atrial flutter.

Digitalis often converts flutter to fibrillation and with the cessation of its administration a normal rhythm may result.

Atrial flutter may be precipitated by cardiac catheterization and other cardiac manoeuvres. It is often not seen in standard lead I.

3. *Atrial fibrillation.* Here the tracing shows no true P waves; these are replaced by oscillations called 'f' waves which are irregular in shape, at a rate of 400 to 600 per min. The ventricular complexes are usually normal, but they occur at irregular intervals which is a characteristic feature giving rise to the typical irregularity of the pulse. Exceptionally, the pulse may be slow and completely regular when complete heart block is associated with atrial fibrillation.

Atrial fibrillation is illustrated in figure 36.

This dysrhythmia occurs most commonly in rheumatic mitral valvular disease, coronary artery disease and hyperthyroidism. It may also occur in clinically normal hearts and in association with cardiotomy and hypothermia. Its onset may decrease cardiac output by as much as 40%.

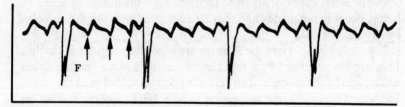

Fig. 35. Atrial flutter.

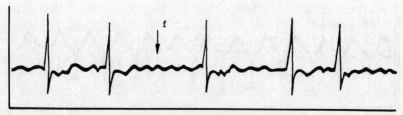

Fig. 36. Atrial fibrillation.

Nodal tachycardia. Here the P wave is usually inverted and the PR interval shortened. The P wave precedes, follows or, occasionally, coincides with the ventricular complex which is usually normal in configuration. Nodal tachycardia is illustrated in figure 37.

When the rate is rapid, e.g. over 200 per min, it is impossible to differentiate nodal from atrial tachycardia and in such instances the term supraventricular tachycardia is applied. Its management is discussed by Sprague (1977) and Donaldson (1979).

Ventricular. Ventricular dysrhythmias are reviewed by Talbot (1979).

1. *Ventricular tachycardia.* This dysrhythmia must always be regarded with apprehension. Here the P waves are lost in the large excursions of the ventricular complexes which have a wide notched appearance. They are regular in rhythm and are followed by large secondary T waves which are directed opposite to the main deflection of the QRS complex. Paroxysmal ventricular tachycardia is illustrated in figure 38.

A form of episodic irregular ventricular tachycardia known as *torsade de pointes* is characterized by a changing QRS axis during the burst of tachycardia and often leads to ventricular fibrillation. It may be associated with hypokalaemia or the prolonged QT interval syndrome.

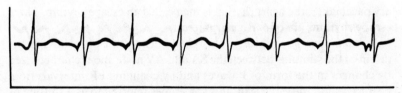

Fig. 37. Nodal tachycardia.

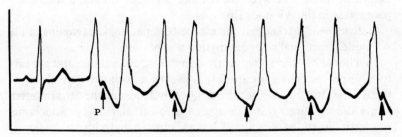

Fig. 38. Paroxysmal ventricular tachycardia.

2. *Ventricular flutter.*   This is very similar to ventricular tachycardia. It is produced by a single ventricular ectopic focus firing at a rate of 200 to 300 per minute and consists of a series of smooth sine waves with absent P and T waves.

3. *Ventricular fibrillation.*   This dysrhythmia is illustrated in figure 33. It occurs when the contractions of individual myocardial fibres are out of phase. Excitation then spreads from one fibre which contracts to another which is resting. This excitation is effective only when the refractory period is abnormally short. It is recognized by its totally irregular appearance which may be coarse or fine. Defibrillation will usually be successful when the ventricular fibrillation is of the coarse variety. Adgey and Webb (1979) discuss management in acute myocardial infarction.

Under normal conditions the long refractory period of cardiac muscle as compared with that of skeletal muscle protects it from fibrillation.

Escape rhythm

When a secondary pacemaker takes over for the occasional cycle the result is an escape beat. This is difficult to distinguish from an extrasystole; the primary difference is that the escape beat is delayed but the extrasystole is premature. If the pacemaker in the SA node is slowed down, for a period a regular cardiac cycle develops fired by the subsidiary pacemaker; the heart rhythm is then called an escape rhythm. Three escape rhythms are of particular interest.

1. *Wandering pacemaker.*   This phenomenon refers to shifts in the origin of the stimulus between the SA and AV node and is characterized by changes in the form of P waves and by changing PR intervals from beat to beat in the same lead. It is sometimes referred to as a shifting or sliding nodal rhythm. Figure 39 illustrates a wandering pacemaker with excursions limited between the SA and AV node (a) and a wandering pacemaker in the AV node (b).

2. *Junctional rhythm.*   If the escape beat pacemaker remains in the AV node, junctional or nodal rhythm is produced.

Junctional rhythm is frequently seen during anaesthesia and appears to have no special significance. It is usually associated with increased vagal tone. It may also occur during stimulation of the atrial musculature during surgery and during cardiac catheterization. Junctional rhythm is illustrated in figure 40. It may be associated with a reduction of cardiac output in the region of 20%.

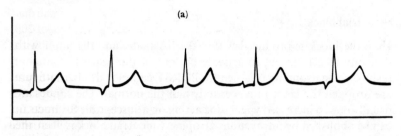

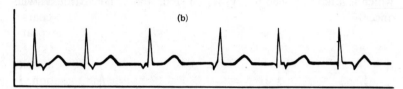

Fig. 39. (a) Wandering pacemaker with excursions limited between the SA and upper AV node. (b) wandering pacemaker in the AV node.

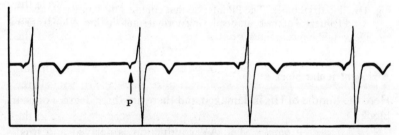

Fig. 40. Junctional (nodal) rhythm.

3. *Ventricular escape rhythm.* This occurs when the rhythm is established by a pacemaker in the ventricle. On rare occasions this is an idioventricular pacemaker with a fast rate but it is more usual for this rhythm to develop in cases of complete AV block (see figure 45). This rhythm may show wide distorted QRS complexes.

HEART BLOCK

This is a condition in which there is a defective conduction in some part of the heart. It is rarely seen in children except with severe low cardiac output states.

Sinoatrial block

Here the block is produced within the SA node, and the impulse has difficulty in getting out to activate the rest of the heart. It commonly results in the dropping of an entire PQRST complex. If alternate beats are dropped the heart rate is exactly half the normal. The condition is usually due to increased vagal tone acting on a susceptible SA node and can be abolished by intravenous atropine. Sinoatrial block is illustrated in figure 41. It is sometimes a manifestation of the sick sinus syndrome which is a term applied to a group of sinus and atrial rhythm disturbances.

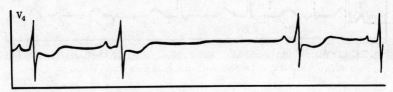

Fig. 41. Sinoatrial block. The PP interval that contains the pause is double the PP interval of the beats displaying normal sinus rhythm. A longer pause would indicate sinus arrest.

Atrioventricular block

Here the bundle of His is damaged and there are three degrees of heart block.

1. *First degree block.* The AV conduction is delayed and this is reflected in a prolongation of the PR interval so that it exceeds 0·2 s (figure 42).

2. *Second degree heart block.* Mobitz has described two types of second degree block. In one type, repeated episodes of progressive lengthening of the PR interval eventually lead to a failure of conduction (figure 43). This is known as the Wenckebach phenomenon or Mobitz type I block. A second type known as Mobitz type II block has a constant PR interval when conduction occurs, but at regular or irregular intervals a P wave is not followed by a QRS complex (figure 44). Type II block is usually associated with more serious disease in the His–Purkinje system.

First and second degree heart block are referred to as partial heart block.

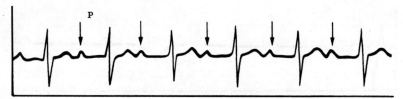

Fig. 42. First degree heart block.

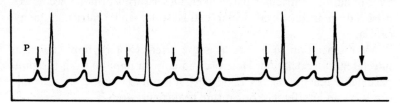

Fig. 43. Second degree heart block (Wenckebach's phenomenon).

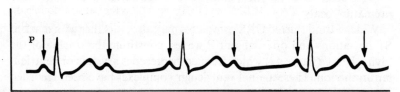

Fig. 44. Second degree (2:1) heart block.

3. *Complete or third degree AV block.* None of the atrial impulses reach the ventricles and so the beats of atria and ventricles are completely dissociated, bearing no relationship to one another. The ventricles beat with an independent rhythm, and at a slower rate—usually less than 40 per min. The independent ventricular beats arise from the most rhythmic part of the ventricle, usually the region of the bundle below the site of the block. The excitation process, therefore, reaches the two ventricles along the normal channel of the two branches of the bundle. The ventricular complex is quite normal in character. This is illustrated in figure 45. Ward and Camm (1979) discuss its management.

Complete or third degree AV block is a non-specific form of AV dissociation, i.e. a rhythm where the atria and ventricles beat independently. The atria are activated by the sinus pacemaker, and the ventricles

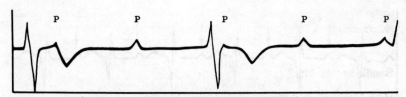

Fig. 45. Third degree (complete) heart block.

by a nodal or ventricular pacemaker. Other forms of non-specific AV dissociation include ventricular extrasystoles and ventricular tachycardia.

AV dissociation in a specific sense refers to a rhythm known as interference dissociation. Here occasionally an impulse from the sinus pacemaker reaches the AV node when it is not in a refractory state and produces an interference or capture beat (figure 46).

If the ventricular pacemaker is located in the bundle branches or in the ventricular muscle (idioventricular rhythm), the QRS complexes are wide, slurred and notched, and have characteristics of ventricular premature beats.

Widened and slurred QRS complexes may also, together with marked ST deviations and often absent P waves, constitute the tracing of the 'dying heart' (figure 47) which frequently precedes asystole or ventricular fibrillation. These agonal ventricular complexes have been recorded

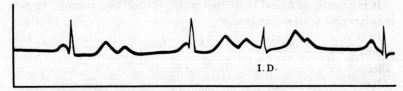

Fig. 46. Interference dissociation. ID: Interference beat (capture beat).

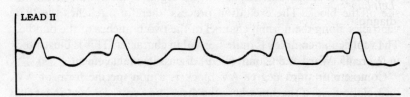

Fig. 47. 'Dying heart' pattern.

up to 45 min after cessation of the heart's contraction and of respiration (Katz and Pick 1956).

Bundle branch block

Here the block occurs in one or other of the bundle branches.

Right bundle branch block (RBBB). When the right bundle is blocked the diagnostic electrocardiographic signs are:

1. QRS widened to 0·12 s or more.
2. Late onset of the intrinsicoid deflection over the right ventricular leads (V1 and V2).
3. Increased amplitude of the R^1 wave in the right precordial leads.
4. Depression of the ST segment and inversion of the T wave (typical block) over the right precordial leads. In atypical block the T wave is upright.
5. Left ventricular precordial leads show a slurred broad S wave due to the late right ventricular depolarization.
6. A QR pattern in lead AVR.
7. Frequently a broad S wave in lead 1.

Right bundle branch block is illustrated in figure 48. Note the R–S–R pattern in leads V1 and V2 sometimes called an rR^1 pattern or an 'M' wave.

It is sometimes found in a heart which is otherwise normal. It then may have no serious significance.

In disease, right bundle branch block is associated with conditions producing great dilatation of the right ventricle, such as atrial septal defects, where it occurs in partial or complete form in 95% of cases.

It may also be associated with pulmonary embolism, coronary artery, and hypertensive and valvular heart disease.

Left bundle branch block (LBBB). When the left bundle is blocked the diagnostic electrocardiographic signs are:

1. QRS widened to 0·12 s or more.
2. Late onset of the intrinsicoid deflection in leads over the left ventricle (V4–V6).
3. Depressed ST segments and inverted T waves over the left precordial leads.

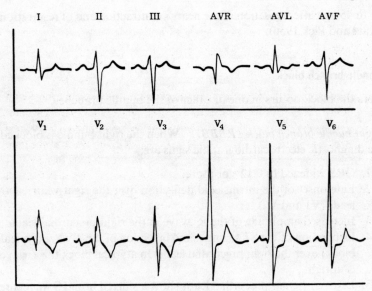

Fig. 48. Right bundle branch block.

4. Right ventricular precordial leads (V1–V3) show a slurred broad S wave due to the late left ventricular depolarization and ST segments may be elevated slightly.

Left bundle branch block is illustrated in figure 49. Very rarely left bundle branch block may be present in a clinically normal heart. It is seen most commonly in coronary artery disease, hypertensive heart disease and aortic stenosis.

Hemiblock

The left bundle branch is now known to have at least two conducting systems. Either of these may show a block when the other does not; this is called hemiblock. Left anterior hemiblock occurs when conduction is interrupted in the anterior-superior division and is characterized by a marked left axis deviation and deep terminal S waves in leads II, III and AVF and a tall R in AVL.

If the posterior-inferior division is blocked then it is called left posterior hemiblock. This produces right axis deviation and a prominent S wave in lead I and AVL and a tall R wave in leads II, III and AVF.

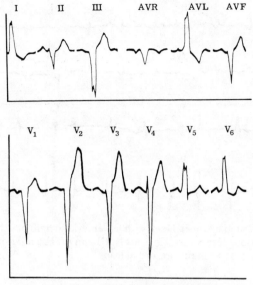

Fig. 49. Left bundle branch block.

The observation of hemiblock can assist in determining the site of myocardial infarction.

RBBB and hemiblock. When this combination occurs the characteristics of RBBB are seen in the precordial leads and the characteristics of the hemiblock in the standard and augmented leads (figure 50).

This combination is frequently seen in the early stage of Lenègre's disease, a degenerative disease of the conducting fibres of the bundle branches. RBBB alone usually occurs first and is then associated with a hemiblock, most frequently left anterior hemiblock.

The risk of RBBB plus hemiblock developing into acute complete heart block during anaesthesia should not be ignored. It has been suggested that the patient be paced prior to the induction of anaesthesia.

Phasic aberrant ventricular conduction

An isolated, bizarre QRS complex is not necessarily the result of an ectopic ventricular discharge but may be due to a temporary bundle branch block following a supraventricular impulse, and has been termed aberrant ventricular conduction. This phenomenon is due to unequal

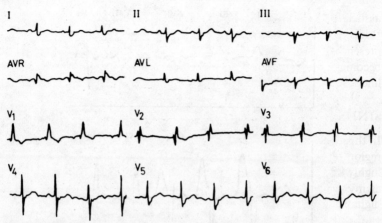

Fig. 50. Right bundle branch block with left anterior hemiblock. Note left axis
deviation, deep S waves in leads II, III and AVF, a tall R in AVL and a
RBBB pattern in the precordial leads.

refractory periods of the bundle branches and is more likely to occur
when the supraventricular impulses are premature. It may be temporary
(phasic) or permanent (non-phasic) (Schamroth and Chester 1963). The
recognition of this conduction defect is important as the differentiation
of supraventricular from ventricular rhythms affects both prognosis and
treatment (Annotation, *Lancet* 1970). For the diagnosis of phasic aberrant ventricular conduction there must be a P wave before, and related
to, the bizarre QRS complex. P waves are best seen in leads II, V1, an
oesophageal, an S5 or an MCL1 lead.

Wolff–Parkinson–White syndrome. This is a pre-excitation anomaly in
which the early part of the QRS complex is disturbed by the premature
activation of the ventricles producing a delta wave which is slurred. The
PR interval is shortened by the delta wave to less than 0·10 s. The
impulse passes through an abnormal lateral muscle band from the atria
to the ventricles called the bundle of Kent. The impulse subsequently
spreading by the normal pathways usually completes the activation of
the ventricles so that every beat is a fusion beat. Although the PR
interval is short the PS interval is normal (figure 51).

There are two types, A and B. In type A the QRS complex is upright in
the precordial leads and indicates a left-sided bundle of Kent; in type B

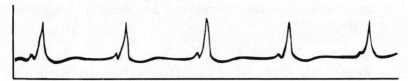

Fig. 51. Wolff-Parkinson-White syndrome.

the QRS complex is negative with a dominant S in the precordial leads and is seen with a right-sided bundle of Kent.

The anomaly may be associated with intractable paroxysmal tachycardia and a negative delta wave which may be confused with a pathological Q wave. Suppan (1979) considers althesin the induction agent of choice in this condition and van der Starre (1978) also discusses its management.

Apart from the bundle of Kent there are two other abnormal atrioventricular communications.

The fibres of Mahaim arise below the AV node and produce a similar QRS pattern to the W–P–W syndrome without a short PR interval.

James' tract produces the L–G–L (Lown–Ganong–Levine) syndrome. This tract by-passes the AV node but re-enters normal conducting pathways at a lower level. The PR interval is short but the QRS complex is normal.

These abnormal pathways are all capable of producing paroxysmal ventricular tachycardia by a re-entry mechanism. (Krikler and Goodwin 1975).

Parasystole.   This is a relatively rare dual rhythm. It consists of simultaneous activity of two independent impulse forming centres one of which is 'protected' from the other, each competing to activate the atria or ventricles or both. The parasystolic pacemaker may be located anywhere in the heart but is commonly located in the ventricles, less commonly in the AV junction and rarely in the atria.

The diagnosis is made by proving the independence of the ectopic rhythm from the basic rhythm by demonstrating varying coupling intervals, constant shortest interectopic intervals and the frequent appearance of fusion beats.

Parasystole is most frequently encountered in elderly patients with arteriosclerotic hypertensive disease and is more frequently seen in males.

Parasystole is resistant to antiarrhythmic drug therapy and may carry a poor prognosis.

Prolonged QT interval syndrome. The normal QT interval should usually be less than 0·43 s. When a much longer QT interval is found in an otherwise normal ECG a case of the prolonged QT interval syndrome should be suspected. It is often associated with congenital deafness and ventricular fibrillation. It provides a very high risk for anaesthesia and it has been suggested that beta blockers should be administered prior to induction (Wig *et al* 1979). Owitz *et al* (1979) discuss the likely effects of a number of anaesthetic agents and demonstrated that a left stellate ganglion block could restore the QT interval to normal.

COMMON ARTEFACTS

Any study of a large series of ECG tracings will reveal occasional peculiar patterns. Many of these can be traced to origins other than the heart of the patient and so are called artefacts. In the operating theatre some unusual artefacts occur and will be discussed in Chapter 5. Some of the more common artefacts are given below.

Muscle tremor. It is important for the conscious patient to be warm and relaxed when the record is taken as any muscle tremor such as that produced by shivering can alter the tracing. This type of interference is illustrated in figure 52. A more marked tremor is seen in Parkinson's disease (Livesley 1973), and also in myoclonus.

Movement of the patient. Movement on the part of the patient with the associated contraction of skeletal muscle causes sudden changes in the potential difference across the electrodes (figure 53).

Shifting of the base or isoelectric line. This is often due to cutaneous currents, polarization of electrodes, variations in cutaneous resistance, disturbance of contact of some electrodes on the body or wires conducting electricity in the vicinity of the recording leads and is illustrated in figure 54.

Loose contacts. These may occur in any part of the circuit and produce sudden shifting of the base line illustrated in figure 55.

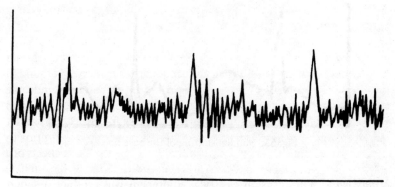

Fig. 52. Muscle tremor.

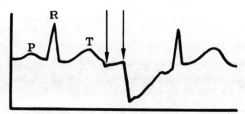

Fig. 53. Movement of the patient.

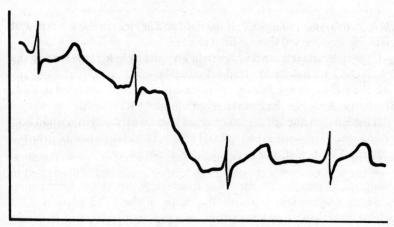

Fig. 54. Shifting of the base line.

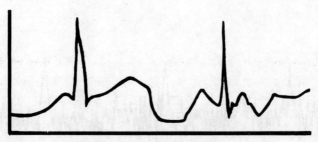

Fig. 55. Sudden shifting of the base line.

Mains hum.   On occasion electrical equipment will produce a signal picked up across the patient of gross interference due to 50-cycle alternating current as shown in figure 56.

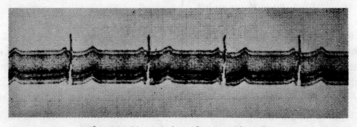

Fig. 56. 50-cycle interference ('hum').

Incorrectly connected leads.   If the right and left legs or the left arm and right leg are reversed there is little change.

If the right and left arms or the right arm and right leg are reversed the P and QRS are inverted in lead I (figure 57).

If the right arm and left leg are reversed P waves are inverted in leads II, III and AVF but the P wave is upright in AVR.

If the left arm and left leg are reversed lead I is identical to normal lead II and lead II is identical to normal lead I. Lead III shows an inverted pattern. AVL is identical to AVF. AVR is not altered.

Faulty ECG machines.   An ECG machine which is not functioning correctly may seriously distort the shape of the ECG pattern. This artefact is difficult to detect except by comparing tracings of the same patient with another machine.

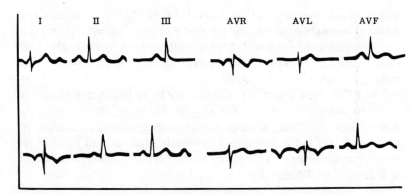

Fig. 57. Upper tracing: Normal ECG picture. Lower tracing: Leads incorrectly connected. Right and left arm leads reversed. Lead I is mirror image of itself, leads II and III are reversed, as are also leads AVR and AVL (Compare with figure 19 which illustrates the ECG in dextrocardia).

Incorrect calibration will produce incorrect heights for the components of the ECG but will otherwise leave the pattern unaffected. As it is normal practice to provide internal standards for calibration such a fault is unpardonable.

Another possible fault particularly with battery machines is that the paper will run at the wrong speed. This can be checked by arranging substantial mains interference and using the 50-cycle wave to calibrate the paper speed.

SYSTEMATIC SCRUTINY OF THE PREOPERATIVE ECG

The anaesthetist faced with a preoperative twelve-lead ECG must scrutinize it with care to ensure that the right steps are taken to ensure the safest possible anaesthetic. Some ECG tracings will yield obvious evidence of a patient at risk; others will only yield their data by a diligent scrutiny. Once the suspicions of the anaesthetist are aroused he may find it desirable to call for the opinion of a cardiologist. The ECG reflects not only the condition of the heart but also the effect of drugs and of some pathological conditions in other parts of the body (Harley 1979).

The following method of conducting a close scrutiny is but one suggested. First examine the main components P, QRS, ST segment, T and U waves, then examine the intervals PR and QT. It is assumed that major abnormalities in rate and the existence of well marked patterns of dysrhythmia will be obvious. Extrasystoles provide considerable difficulty as infrequent ones may not reveal themselves in the short strips of tracing provided.

The ECG signs are only presented briefly and reference should be made to the earlier part of the chapter for more details and fuller descriptions of the pathological conditions. Suggestions as to cause are the most likely but different ECG anomalies may not all point in the same direction; experience together with other patient data must be used to make the final diagnosis.

P wave

1. Prominent in leads II and V1: atrial hypertrophy.
2. Inverted P waves in standard leads: junctional (nodal) rhythm.
3. Inverted P wave in lead I only: dextrocardia or incorrect placement of electrodes.
4. Absent P wave; sick sinus syndrome, hyperkalaemia or AV nodal rhythm.

QRS complex

Right ventricular pattern in lateral precordial leads: clockwise rotation. Left ventricular pattern in right precordial leads: counter clockwise rotation.

1. Low voltage in all leads: myxoedema, thick chest wall, emphysema, anasarca, pericardial effusion, myocardial infarction and CO poisoning.
2. High voltage in all leads: ventricular hypertrophy, thin chest wall, hypertension, and hyperthyroidism.
3. Slurred and widened complexes in the precordial leads: bundle branch block.
4. Positive QRS in lead I and negative QRS lead III: left axis deviation. Negative in lead I and positive in lead III: right axis deviation.
5. Deep S in leads II, III and AVF and a tall R in AVL: left anterior hemiblock.
6. Deep Q waves: transmural infarction.
7. Tall R waves in V1 and V2: true posterior infarction.

ST segment

1. ST elevation (Pardee curve); myocardial infarction; elevated and concave upwards: pericarditis.
2. Depressed concave upward ST segments in V1 and V2: true posterior infarction.
3. The mirror image of a correction mark or saucer-shaped depression with concavity upwards: digitalis effect.
4. ST depression with convexity upwards: ventricular hypertrophy with 'strain'.

T wave

1. Low or inverted: myocardial ischaemia; hypokalaemia.
2. Tall and tented: hyperkalaemia.
3. Tall symmetrical T waves in V1 and V2 true posterior infarction.
4. Inverted in typical bundle branch block: digitalis and hypertension.

U wave

1. Prominent: hypokalaemia.
2. Inverted: myocardial ischaemia and hypertension.

PR interval

1. Prolonged: myocardial ischaemia; digitalis; first degree heart block; hyperkalaemia.
2. Shortened: junctional (nodal) rhythm, atrial extrasystole and W–P–W syndrome.
3. Varying: Wenckebach phenomenon.
4. Dissociated: complete heart block.

QT interval

1. Prolonged: myocardial infarction; cerebral injury; drug effects (hypocalcaemia; hypokalaemia; quinidine; procaine amide); prolonged QT interval syndrome.
2. Shortened: Drug effects (hypercalcaemia; digitalis).

DYSRHYTHMIAS

The rhythm observed should be compared with figures 28–49. One of the most important ways of distinguishing between dysrhythmias is the behaviour of the P wave relative to the QRS complex. The P wave is usually best seen in leads II or V1.

Example

Figure 58 is the preoperative tracing of a middle-aged male patient who is under treatment for hypertension. Systematic scrutiny reveals sinus rhythm at a rate of 80 beats per min. The P waves are tall and wide in standard leads II and III and in lead AVF. In lead V1 the P wave is biphasic. The P wave changes suggest left atrial hypertrophy.

The QRS configuration is normal but there is a markedly increased voltage suggesting hypertension.

The T wave in the standard leads is inverted and there is a typical downward sloping ST segment with the convexity upwards and an inverted T wave in lead V6 which suggests left ventricular hypertrophy with a 'strain' pattern.

The PR interval in standard lead II is 0·24 s suggesting first degree heart block.

The systematic scrutiny of this patient's preoperative tracing accordingly suggests that he has left atrial hypertrophy, first degree heart block and left ventricular hypertrophy.

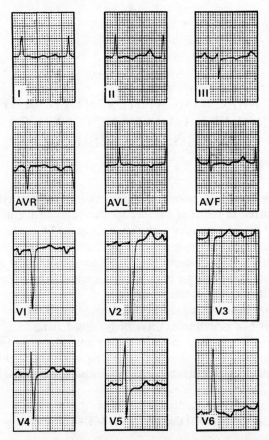

Fig. 58. This is the twelve-lead ECG of a middle-aged hypertensive male who is not responding well to the drug treatment for his hypertension.

4

THE EFFECT OF ANAESTHETIC AGENTS, ELECTROLYTE IMBALANCE AND CARDIAC DRUGS ON THE ECG

In Chapters 1 to 3, the nature of the normal and abnormal ECG has been considered in terms of the electrophysiology of the heart. Drugs which affect the heart may produce changes in the ECG and this is true whether the drugs are being given as medicine or as part of an anaesthetic procedure. This chapter considers effects produced by drugs likely to be met within anaesthesia but must be regarded as only one section of a study of ECGs and pharmacology.

The major action of drugs is to cause dysrhythmias. In the last chapter the aetiology of dysrhythmias was briefly considered.

Electrolyte imbalance may occur during anaesthesia and so its ECG effects are discussed. Cardiac drugs are frequently used before, during and after operation and so their effects are also summarized.

SIGNIFICANCE OF DYSRHYTHMIAS

ECG studies during anaesthesia have shown a very common occurrence of dysrhythmia ranging from 10% to over 80%. Clearly few of these dysrhythmias can be very significant or the administration of any anaesthetic would be highly dangerous.

In reading reports of ECG studies under anaesthesia, it is important to examine findings on dysrhythmias closely to see whether in fact those reported are clinically significant. One list of major dysrhythmias (Rollason and Dundas 1970) is as follows:

1. Prolonged bursts of unifocal ventricular extrasystoles.
2. Multifocal ventricular extrasystoles.
3. Ventricular tachycardia.
4. Pulsus bigeminus.

PREMEDICATION

Apart from the sinus tachycardia usually produced by such drugs as atropine and chlorpromazine, routine premedication appears to have no significant effect on the ECG in the healthy subject. As the main coronary inflow occurs in diastole, drugs which increase the heart rate shorten diastole and should be avoided in patients with hyperthyroidism and cardiac disease, except those with heart block.

Apprehension and anxiety are common causes of tachycardia and should be dealt with by appropriate reassurance and sedation. The barbiturates and tranquillizers appear to produce no significant ECG changes in normal dosage. Indeed diazepam is reputed to have antidysrhythmic properties.

Morphia and scopolamine

Kurtz *et al* (1936) studied premedication with these agents and found a tendency to produce small changes in the QRS complex and T wave together with slight ST depression and an increase in pulse rate.

Atropine

In the conscious and fit patient intravenous atropine may produce a tachycardia or a bradycardia (Rollason 1957, Thomas 1965). Large doses accelerate and small doses slow the heart rate. Rapid injection tends to produce tachycardia and ECG changes (Gottlieb and Sweet 1963). The drug may produce a supraventricular dysrhythmia such as nodal rhythm and nodal extrasystoles (Averil and Lamb 1959, Jones *et al* 1961), and in the presence of adrenaline, CO_2 retention and electrolyte imbalance, it may precipitate ventricular fibrillation. It may predispose to a multifocal ventricular dysrhythmia in patients anaesthetized with cyclopropane and halothane, and in patients subjected to topical analgesia with cocaine (Orr and Jones 1967).

The routine use of atropine premedication should be avoided especially for the dysrhythmic effects produced (Mirakhur *et al* 1978).

Other drugs

These include pethidine, the antihistamines, the phenothiazines and the neuroleptic agents. They have however, produced no significant ECG changes in normal dosage in the fit patient provided respiratory depression and CO_2 retention are avoided. Neuroleptic analgesia, however, does not protect the patient from reflexes which predispose to cardiac dysrhythmia (Eerola *et al* 1963), but it can block the pressor response to intubation (Rollason and Emslie 1972).

INDUCTION AGENTS

Barbiturates

Thiopentone may cause an increase in the height of the P wave, but this is probably related to an increase in pulse rate and a fall in BP rather than to the drug *per se* (Rollason and Hough 1958).

Pre-existing ventricular extrasystoles may be abolished by both thiopentone and methohexitone.

While sinus tachycardia may occur during the ultra-light methohexitone technique used in chairside dentistry, it is unusual to observe any significant ECG changes except in the very nervous patients (Rollason and Dundas 1970).

Propanidid

This intravenous induction agent is a eugenol derivative marketed under the name of Epontol. Apart from an occasional tachycardia no significant ECG changes have been observed when the drug is injected slowly (Wynands and Burfoot 1965, Rollason and Dundas 1970). Changes, however, e.g. various forms of heart block, have been recorded when the drug is injected rapidly and a brief antidysrhythmic action has been demonstrated (Johnstone and Barron 1968). This antidysrhythmic property is illustrated in figure 59.

Diazepam

This benzodiazepine derivative is marketed under the name of Valium. No significant ECG changes have been observed although an occasional vagotonic reaction has been noted when used in the high dosage necessary to induce unconsciousness in the unpremedicated patient (Rollason 1968, 1970).

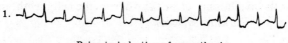

Prior to induction of anaesthesia

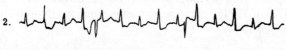

After insertion of needle

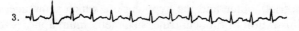

After induction with propanidid (450 mg)

Fig. 59. Antidysrhythmic effect of propanidid in 34-year-old female weight 70 kg (lead I).

Gamma-hydroxybutyrate

The only recorded ECG change with this agent has been sinus bradycardia during induction (Solway and Sadove 1965), but this does not occur when no other drug has been given beforehand.

Hypnomidate (etomidate)

This new intravenous agent can be irritant to the vein wall and cause muscle movements but it does not appear to produce any ECG changes.

Ketalar

This is the trade name for ketamine hydrochloride which is a rapid acting non-barbiturate general anaesthetic for intravenous and intramuscular use. It produces a transient significant increase of both systolic and diastolic blood pressures but no ECG changes have been recorded. Indeed it is reputed to have antidysrhythmic properties. Johnstone (1976) has shown it to be a direct myocardial stimulant acting by increasing the availability of calcium across the cell membranes of the myocardial and Purkinje systems.

Althesin

This steroid intravenous induction agent has produced no ECG changes (Campbell *et al* 1971) and appears to have antidysrhythmic properties (Rollason *et al* 1974).

MUSCLE RELAXANTS

Apart from sinus tachycardia and occasional dysrhythmias produced by gallamine triethiodide and the hypotension, which sometimes follows the administration of tubocurarine, suxamethonium appears to be the only relaxant which produces significant ECG changes in the absence of hypoxia and CO_2 retention. Tubocurarine is a myocardial depressant being a calcium-ion antagonist (Johnston *et al* 1978).

The non-depolarizing relaxants, alcuronium and pancuronium bromide are virtually devoid of cardiovascular side effects and no ECG changes have been observed.

Suxamethonium

This relaxant when given intravenously can not only produce a simple sinus bradycardia but also dysrhythmias in both adults and children (Leigh *et al* 1957). The nature of the dysrhythmia is a depression of excitation and conduction of the cardiac impulse producing changes in the P wave, PR interval, QRS complex and asystole lasting over 20 s (McLeskey *et al* 1978). These changes are illustrated in figure 60.

Cases of prolonged cardiac arrest following the injection of suxamethonium in a severely burned patient have been reported by Allen *et al* (1961), Bush (1964) and Tolmie *et al* (1967).

Suxamethonium should be avoided in the burned patient during the period from the ninth to the sixtieth day after the burn. Electrolyte imbalance may already exist and suxamethonium by increasing the serum potassium may precipitate a cardiac arrest. It should also be avoided in cases of traumatic paraplegia and major muscle injury.

A second dose of suxamethonium may produce a severe bradycardia but this response can be blocked by atropine and prevented by the prior administration of tubocurarine, alcuronium, gallamine and pancur-

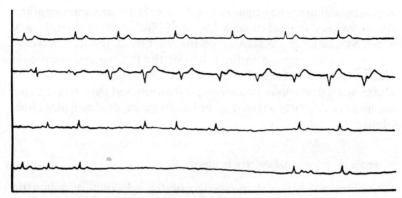

Fig. 60. Top tracing: Variations of the P wave. Second tracing: Wide QRS complexes followed by inverted P waves. Third tracing: Wenckebach's phenomenon. Bottom tracing: Asystole.

onium in quantities of one-quarter or less of their muscle relaxant level (Mathias *et al* 1970).

The administration of suxamethonium to the fully digitalized patient can produce dangerous ventricular dysrhythmias and these dysrhythmias can be abolished by the injection of tubocurarine. In the partially digitalized patient it produces changes characteristic of digitalization.

Suxamethonium should be used with care in the patient who is receiving quinidine as this alkaloid has a depressant effect on skeletal as well as cardiac muscle. It acts both directly on the muscle fibre and on neuromuscular transmission at the motor end plate and prolonged apnoea may follow (Grogono 1963).

The action of suxamethonium can be prolonged by tacrine hydrochloride but no ECG changes have been associated with the latter agent.

INHALATIONAL AGENTS

The effect of these on the ECG varies. Some, like nitrous oxide, in the presence of adequate oxygenation and ventilation produce no effects whereas others like chloroform and cyclopropane may produce dangerous dysrhythmias.

The changes are due to either vagal stimulation or sympathetic activity or a combination of both. Vagal stimulation results in a bradycardia with a reduction in the height of the P wave. If the stimulus is marked and unopposed, partial or complete heart block or even asystole may occur. Sympathetic overactivity, on the other hand, results in a tachycardia, with an increase in the height of the P wave and occasional ventricular extrasystoles. If the stimulus is marked and unopposed the ventricular extrasystoles become more frequent and may develop into the multifocal variety which may be the precursor of ventricular fibrillation.

Anaesthetic agents and catecholamines

Catecholamines have a marked effect on the behaviour of automatic cells and so are responsible for many dysrhythmias. Many anaesthetic agents sensitize the heart to the effect of catecholamines. Anaesthetic agents which produce this sensitizing effect include trichlorethylene, ethyl chloride, cyclopropane, halothane and chloroform. Adrenergic agents which are capable of producing dysrhythmias in the presence of cyclopropane or halogenated hydrocarbons include adrenaline, noradrenaline and metaraminol. Some adrenergic agents including ephedrine, phenylephrine, methoxamine and mephentermine rarely produce dysrhythmias when used with these agents (Foex 1977).

Chloroform

The classical work of Hill (1931a,b) demonstrated multifocal ventricular tachycardia in about 50% of cases during induction and the dysrhythmia disappeared as anaesthesia was deepened.

The liberation of endogenous adrenaline from the suprarenal by fear, pain, hypoxia, CO_2 retention or the injection of adrenaline by the surgeon may act on a chloroform-sensitized myocardium to precipitate a dangerous or even fatal ventricular dysrhythmia.

Vagal stimulation may also be the cause of death (Waters 1951).

With all precautions cardiac arrest can occasionally occur (Hart and Duthie 1964). Griffiths (1979) however, claims that when used to produce only unconsciousness, analgesia and areflexia, it is safe and devoid of ECG changes.

Ethyl chloride

This agent should be treated with the same respect as chloroform for its administration carries similar risks and its use is now restricted to the production of localized refrigeration analgesia.

Trichlorethylene

Almost every known form of cardiac dysrhythmia has been reported during anaesthesia with this agent.

It is now, however, only used as an analgesic supplement and provided hypoxia and CO_2 retention do not occur and adrenaline is avoided dysrhythmias in these light levels of anaesthesia are rarely observed.

Should higher concentrations be inadvertently used tachypnoea and CO_2 retention occur with the resultant appearance of ventricular dysrhythmias, but these can be abolished by the intravenous injection of pethidine (Johnstone 1951).

Diethyl ether

From a practical point of view this agent is probably still the safest, although deliberate forced inflation of the lungs with a high concentration of vapour may so stimulate the pulmocardiac reflex that asystole results. This is more likely to occur when the larynx has been paralysed by a relaxant.

Only minor dysrhythmias occur with this agent and adrenaline may safely be used in normal dosage.

Halothane

Halothane remains the most widely used inhalational anaesthetic.

The vagal effects of this agent are common. If the heart rate falls to 40 beats per min it should be corrected by the intravenous injection of 0·15 mg of atropine sulphate, which should be repeated if necessary.

Sympathetic effects also occur. Ventricular extrasystoles are common if CO_2 retention is allowed (Black *et al* 1959, Fukushima *et al* 1968). Ventricular extrasystoles of the multifocal variety and ventricular tachycardia have been seen in the absence of CO_2 retention and hypoxia in light planes of anaesthesia (Rollason and Dundas 1970).

Occasionally intubation under halothane has produced a ventricular dysrhythmia, while stretching of the anal sphincter may produce a similar effect.

The sensitization of the heart to adrenaline by halothane has widely been observed. Ventricular extrasystoles and ventricular tachycardia are common. Cases of cardiac arrest have been reported (Rosen and Roe 1963, de Lange 1963); these seem to have been due to the accidental intravenous injection of adrenaline. In the presence of halothane the injection of adrenaline should either be avoided (Davies 1965), or restricted to the subcutaneous tissues and injected in a concentration not exceeding 1 in 100 000, at a rate not exceeding 1 ml per min (0·01 mg) up to a maximum of 10 ml, in the adult under continuous ECG control (Katz and Katz 1966). In the baby volumes up to 5 ml of 1 in 200 000 produce no ECG changes in paediatric plastic procedures.

As halothane both increases vagal tone and myocardial sensitization to catecholamines, sympathetic stimulation from any cause will facilitate the development of cardiac dysrhythmia even in the presence of adequate oxygenation and ventilation. These dysrhythmias, however, can now be controlled effectively by the use of the cardioselective beta blocker, practolol (Rollason and Hall, 1973). Examples are illustrated in figure 61 (a), (b) and (c). Metoprolol is equally effective (Rollason and Russell 1979).

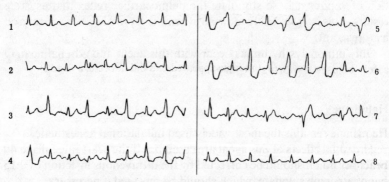

Fig. 61(a). 30-year-old fit male, weight 70·0 kg. As the dysrhythmia was persistent practolol was injected i.v. slowly at 6. Following a dose of 5 mg the dysrhythmia disappeared and did not return (lead I).

It is interesting to note that deep halothane anaesthesia has been used successfully for the surgical removal of a phaeochromocytoma without the appearance of any dysrhythmia (Rollason 1964). Moreover, it has been used for open cardiac surgery during which intracardiac adrenaline was used but no ventricular tachycardia or fibrillation ensued (Orton

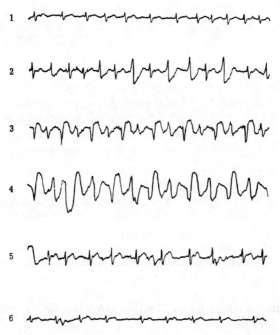

Fig. 61(b). 37-year-old fit female, weight 72·5 kg. As the dysrhythmia was persistent, practolol was injected slowly at 4. Following a dose of 8 mg the dysrhythmia disappeared and did not return (lead I).

and Morris 1959, Dawson *et al* 1960). Nevertheless, the intrusion of frequent ventricular extrasystoles into the ECG pattern should be regarded by the anaesthetist as a warning signal not to be ignored and practolol or metoprolol should be available. Atropine should also be at hand to correct any bradycardia or hypotension should they occur.

The injection of adrenaline and CO_2 retention are however, not the only causes of ventricular dysrhythmias under halothane. Other causes include hypoxia, hypovolaemia, electrolyte imbalance, metabolic acidosis, the intravenous use of atropine and sensory stimulation under light anaesthesia.

Halothane in association with controlled ventilation can produce profound hypotension and this has deliberately and successfully been employed without any significant ECG changes for radical surgery in malignant disease of the face (Robinson 1967), but a very high alveolar

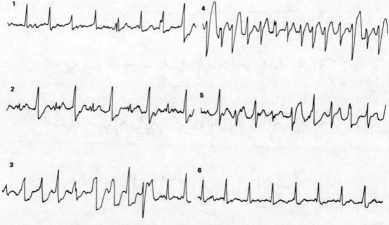

Fig. 61(c). 46-year-old fit male, weight 65·0 kg. As the dysrhythmia was persistent practolol was injected i.v. slowly at 4. Following a dose of 6 mg
the dysrhythmia disappeared and did not return (lead I).

oxygen tension is mandatory if cardiac arrest is to be avoided as cardiac
output is very low.

Halothane facilitates the induction of moderate hypothermia and
does not increase the incidence of ventricular dysrhythmias, provided
the temperature does not fall below 28°C (82·4°F) and good oxygenation and ventilation are ensured (Rollason and Latham 1963).

Methoxyflurane

This fluorinated ether, in its cardiovascular effects, resembles halothane
rather than ether but does not sensitize the heart to adrenaline (Hudon
1961). No characteristic ECG changes have been reported in man.

Fluoromar (fluroxene)

This agent does not appear to sensitize the heart to adrenaline nor to
produce dysrhythmias (Eikard and Skovsted 1975).

Enflurane

This halogenated compound does not appear to produce dysrhythmias

(Egilmez and Dobkin 1972), but the sensitization of the heart to adrenaline by enflurane has been observed (Reisner and Lippmann 1975).

Cyclopropane

This is the only gaseous agent which can produce serious dysrhythmias.

Ventricular dysrhythmias are common in the lighter and deeper levels of cyclopropane anaesthesia in the presence of CO_2 retention, and are further accentuated when an elevated PCO_2 is suddenly reduced, and this is particularly so in the presence of the higher blood concentrations of cyclopropane. Price *et al* (1958), however, have found that bilateral stellate ganglion blockage with a local anaesthetic can render CO_2 retention relatively ineffective in producing these ventricular dysrhythmias. In the patient under cyclopropane anaesthesia, an injection of gallamine may precipitate a ventricular tachycardia and this relaxant should be avoided (Walts and Prescott 1965). The dysrhythmias associated with gallamine are due to sympathomimetic properties in addition to its well-known atropine-like action (Brown and Crout 1968).

Intravenous atropine should also be avoided (Kristoffersen and Clausen 1967).

The incidence of cardiac dysrhythmias during a straight cyclopropane anaesthetic is significantly higher than in a thiopentone–cyclopropane sequence (Seuffert and Urbach 1967).

OTHER DRUGS USED DURING ANAESTHESIA

Adrenaline and noradrenaline

The action of catecholamines on the behaviour of pacemakers has already been discussed. These particular catecholamines are sensitized by inhalational agents like halothane and cyclopropane. Major dysrhythmias are likely to occur including ventricular fibrillation, particularly, if hypoxia, hypercarbia or electrolyte imbalance are present or if cocaine has been used topically. In the presence, however, of persistent ventricular dysrhythmia practolol or metoprolol should be used. This is most likely to occur in a patient with hyperthyroidism or with a phaeochromocytoma. In the latter instance, and in cases of accidental overdosage with adrenaline, phentolamine or phenoxybenzamine should be used in addition to practolol or metoprolol, i.e. alpha and beta blockade.

ECG changes recorded during infusions of adrenaline and noradrenaline include depression of the ST segment, depression and inversion of the T wave and elevation of the U wave (Lepeschkin *et al* 1960).

Adrenaline and noradrenaline should be replaced by felypressin (Octapressin) as this agent has been found to be a safe and effective local vasoconstrictor and its use during cyclopropane, trichlorethylene and halothane anaesthesia does not produce cardiac dysrhythmias. Furthermore, it is safe to use in patients who are on tricyclic antidepressants. A readily available solution is 3% prilocaine which contains 0·03 iu felypressin per ml (Goldman *et al* 1970).

Ergometrine

Although generally considered to be an antidysrhythmic drug, nodal rhythm, a wandering pacemaker and occasional ventricular ectopic activity have been recorded after intravenous use (Baillie 1969a, b).

Syntocinon

In addition to constricting the uterus this drug appears to have antidysrhythmic properties.

Atropine

Although this drug has been discussed in relation to premedication it is referred to again here. After injection it usually produces a triple response: vagal stimulation, vagal imbalance and vagolysis.

To correct a bradycardia, e.g. after suxamethonium or a beta blocker, it should be injected in incremental doses of 0·15 mg i.v. to prevent an overshoot. This is especially important if the bradycardia is associated with pre-existing cardiac disease in the patient as a fatal result may ensue (Massumi *et al* 1972). It is generally accepted that atropine tends to increase the incidence of dysrhythmias in anaesthesia (Eikard and Sorensen 1976, Leighton and Sanders 1976, Eikard and Anderson 1977).

As it is a potentially lethal drug it should only be given when specifically indicated. In some circumstances glycopyrronium may be a more acceptable substitute (Mirakhur *et al* 1978) as it produces no significant ECG changes in therapeutic dosage (Mirakhur 1979).

The diverse ECG changes associated with atropine have been comprehensively reviewed by Shutt and Bowes (1979).

Neostigmine and atropine

These drugs continue to be used routinely to reverse the effect of curarization produced by non-depolarizing relaxants. Some inject the drugs together while others precede the administration of neostigmine by an injection of atropine. Usually no significant ECG changes are seen after either technique when the patient has been well oxygenated and ventilated (Salem *et al* 1970). In the presence of CO_2 retention, secondary to hypoventilation, ECG changes occur which involve most components of the ECG and include extrasystoles, heart block, gross voltage reduction and transient asystole. It would appear that in healthy patients the heart is protected from the effects of neostigmine by a respiratory alkalosis.

The view has been expressed (Pooler 1957) that atropine in association with CO_2 retention is the cause of sudden deaths following the simultaneous intravenous injection of neostigmine and atropine. This view is further substantiated by the fact that sudden deaths have occurred after the injection of atropine alone, before neostigmine was administered, at the end of abdominal operations for obstructive conditions in patients with electrolyte imbalance, tachycardia and CO_2 retention.

Carbon dioxide

Carbon dioxide accumulation during anaesthesia in association with hypoxia, electrolyte imbalance, atropine and adrenaline may predispose to ventricular fibrillation. It should also be remembered that the sudden reduction of a high CO_2 retention may predispose to dangerous ventricular dysrhythmias.

The intraperitoneal insufflation of CO_2 gas to facilitate laparoscopy under general anaesthesia may provoke ventricular dysrhythmias (Scott and Julian 1972), but these can be prevented by adequate positive pressure ventilation (Gordon *et al* 1972).

Amyl nitrite

This agent, which is sometimes used to terminate hiccup during anaesthesia, may produce both a tachycardia and a reversal of direction of the T wave.

Edrophonium chloride (Tensilon)

While useful in the differential diagnosis of a prolonged apnoea follow-ing the use of muscle relaxants, this agent may produce asystole if used to treat paroxysmal supraventricular tachycardias (Youngberg 1979).

ELECTROLYTE IMBALANCE

In the cardiac cell the transmembrane voltage is maintained by a differ-ence in the ionic concentration inside and outside the cell; the depolari-zation and repolarization cycle of the cell depends on the movements of ions across the membrane. Thus changes in the concentration of the different ions are very likely to affect cell behaviour and so cause dysrhythmias. The most important ions present are those of potassium, sodium and calcium.

Potassium

A high serum potassium (hyperkalaemia) may be found in patients with Addison's disease, uraemia, shock, hypoxia, dehydration, severe burns and patients on low sodium diets. It may also be seen in those receiving massive blood transfusions and in those on a potassium chloride drip, particularly in the presence of inadequate renal function. Hyperkalae-mia is characterized initially by tall peaked T waves which may be higher than the QRS complex. These are illustrated in figure 62.

A low serum potassium (hypokalaemia) may be seen in patients with diabetic acidosis, primary aldosteronism, potassium-losing nephritis, excessive diarrhoea, and following the excessive use of steroids and certain diuretics. Hypokalaemia is characterized initially with prolonga-tion of the QT interval, lowering or inversion of the T waves, and prominent U waves. These are illustrated in figure 63. The changes are best seen in lead V4.

Sodium

The variations in plasma sodium concentration normally encountered produce negligible effects on the ECG.

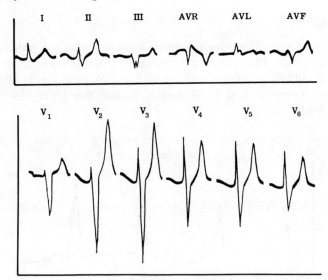

Fig. 62. Hyperkalaemia: serum K 7·6 mEq/litre—a case of uraemia.

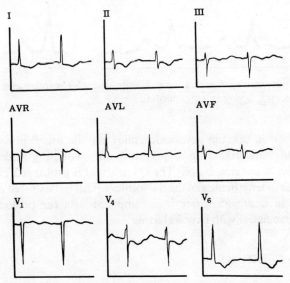

Fig. 63. Hypokalaemia: serum K 1·7 mEq/litre—a case of chronic nephritis. Note depression of ST segments and T waves, prolonged QT and prominent U waves especially in V4.

Calcium

A high serum calcium (hypercalcaemia) may be associated with hyper-parathyroidism. The QT interval varies inversely with the calcium level of the blood and in patients with a parathyroid tumour the QT interval may be so shortened that the ST segment is abolished. This is illustrated in figure 64.

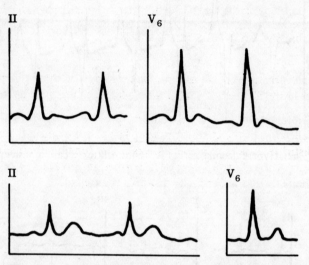

Fig. 64. Upper tracing: hypercalcaemia. Note absent ST segment and short QT interval. Lower tracing: normal.

A low serum calcium (hypocalcaemia) may be found in hypopara-thyroidism, uraemia, after hyperventilation, vomiting and massive transfusion of citrated blood. The QT interval is prolonged but this is mainly due to lengthening of the ST segment. This is illustrated diagram-matically in figure 65 where it is compared with the prolonged QT interval associated with hypokalaemia.

CARDIAC DRUGS

Digitalis

This is the 'great imitator' and is to the ECG what syphilis has been to

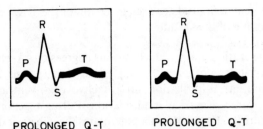

Fig. 65. Left tracing: hypocalcaemia (QT prolongation due to a lengthened ST segment). Right tracing: hypokalaemia (QT prolongation due to a low broad T wave).

medicine. Digitalis in therapeutic dosage most commonly produces changes in the ST segment and T wave. These changes are as follows:

1. Depression of the ST segment in those leads in which the main deflection of the QRS is upright. The shape of the ST segment is distinctive and appears as a straight line running obliquely downwards (the mirror image of a correction mark: $\vee$) or saucer-shaped with the concavity upwards (figure 66).

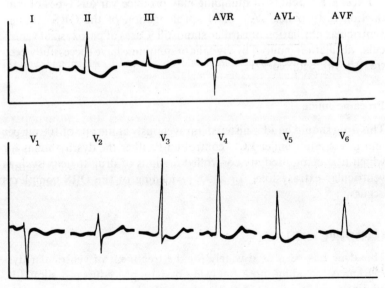

Fig. 66. Digitalis effect.

2. Decrease in amplitude or even inversion of the T wave.
3. Shortening of the QT interval.

Overdigitalization may produce various degrees of AV block, ventricular extrasystoles—often with coupled rhythm (pulsus bigeminus), nodal rhythm, atrial fibrillation, atrial tachycardia, ventricular tachycardia and, rarely, ventricular fibrillation. Pulsus bigeminus is illustrated in figure 31. Hypokalaemia potentiates the effects of digitalis and its correction with intravenous potassium chloride can terminate a digitalis-induced dysrhythmia.

Deutsch and Dalen (1969) have discussed the use of prophylactic digitalization in the preparation of certain patients for anaesthesia and surgery.

Quinidine

ECG changes associated with therapeutic doses of quinidine are:

1. Prolongation of the QT interval.
2. Decrease in the amplitude or even inversion of the T wave.
3. ST segment depression.

Excessive amounts of quinidine may produce various types of conduction disturbances, AV block, prolongation of the QRS interval, ventricular fibrillation or cardiac standstill. Cases of paroxysmal ventricular fibrillation induced by digitalis or quinidine have successfully been treated with beta blockers.

Procaine amide

This drug should be administered intravenously at the rate of 100 mg per min in the adult under ECG control until either the dysrhythmias for which it is being used are controlled or signs of drug toxicity such as ventricular extrasystoles, or a 50% widening of the QRS complexes occur.

Lignocaine

This drug has been used widely for the treatment of ventricular dysrhythmias including those following by-pass procedures. It should be administered in a dose of 1 to 2 mg per kg body weight at a rate not less than 1 mg per min in the same way as procaine amide and with the same precautions. Like procaine amide it may on occasion provoke ventricular tachycardia and fibrillation.

This drug is also used to produce intravenous regional analgesia in Bier's technique. Dysrhythmias including a case of cardiac asystole have followed the removal of the tourniquet (Kennedy *et al* 1965). This is illustrated in figure 67. Prilocaine appears to be devoid of these dangers.

The pain of angina decubitus has successfully been relieved by the

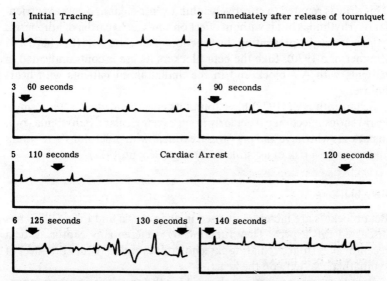

Fig. 67. Asystole following release of tourniquet after i.v. regional analgesia using 0·5% lignocaine and immediate response to external cardiac massage.

thoracic epidural injection of carbonated lignocaine (Bromage 1967) and this resulted in an improvement in the ECG pattern. The attacks of pain were associated with a rapid thready pulse and flattened or inverted T waves but following epidural block of the first four thoracic segments the pulse slowed and the T waves returned to normal.

Isoprenaline

This drug increases the heart rate and stroke volume. It reduces peripheral vascular resistance, dilates the bronchial tree and does not cause potassium release from the liver. It is the drug of choice in the treatment of complete heart block occurring during open cardiac surgery and following myocardial infarction. As an emergency measure it should be infused intravenously (2 mg in 500 ml of 5% dextrose) under ECG control while arrangements are made for pacemaking.

Isoprenaline may cause a transient inversion of the T wave.

Verapamil

This drug is reputed to effectively inhibit ventricular and supraventricular dysrhythmias but is without effect on sinus tachycardia of adrenergic origin. It acts by preventing the function of calcium ions (Brichard and Zimmerman 1970). Like the beta blockers its use is contraindicated in patients with AV block and in the undigitalized patients with heart failure.

Schamroth *et al* (1972) have found its effect immediate after a single intravenous injection particularly in supraventricular dysrhythmias but, in patients who have had previous treatment with practolol, there would appear to be a risk of asystole occurring (Benaim 1972).

Beta blockers

Beta blockers are increasingly used in anaesthesia and Foëx (1977) has discussed this aspect. They function by preferentially capturing beta receptor sites from circulating catecholamines and so reduce the effect of sympathetic activity on the heart.

Beta blockers are particularly used for the prevention and treatment of dysrhythmias arising from laryngoscopy, bronchoscopy, administration of catecholamines and hypercapnoea. They are used to prevent the tachycardia associated with the use of induced hypotension and to suppress dysrhythmias during induced hypothermia. Beta blockers can be used to prevent the hypertensive response to sympathetic stimulation; these hypertensive responses can be particularly severe in patients suffering from arterial hypertension or ischaemic heart disease.

Beta blockers interact with anaesthetic agents. Such blockers which lack sympathomimetic activity have only a small depressant effect on the cardiovascular system under halothane or halothane nitrous oxide anaesthesia. With trichlorethylene, methoxyflurane, enflurane, cyclopropane and ether anaesthesia the effect is large and potentially hazardous.

The beta blockers most frequently used in anaesthesia are practolol and metoprolol and these are cardioselective.

Vaughan-Williams (1970) has divided drugs like the beta blockers which possess antidysrhythmic activity into four classes and these are illustrated in Table 2.

Table 2. Drugs having antidysrhythmic activity

Class I Slowing of rate of rise of depolarization	Class II Antisympathetic	Class III Prolongation of action potential	Class IV Calcium antagonism
Procaine amide	Beta blockers	Procaine amide	Verapamil
Lignocaine		Bretylium	Tubocurarine
Beta blockers		Beta blockers	Beta blockers

Targets in antidysrhythmic therapy (Krikler 1974) are illustrated in figure 68. The aim is twofold: (a) to diminish increased automaticity, and (b) to interrupt a re-entry mechanism.

Diminished automaticity may be achieved by:

1. Slowing the rate of rise of spontaneous diastolic depolarization (figure 68a).
2. Increasing the threshold potential (figure 68b).
3. Prolonging the refractory period by increasing the duration of the action potential (figure 68c).
4. Lowering the maximum repolarization potential at the end of phase 3.

Re-entry may be blocked by prolonging the circuit time within the AV node until conduction is too slow to support it (figure 68d).

Antidysrhythmic drugs like the beta blockers may act in more than one of these ways.

Occasionally a tachydysrhythmia which proves refractory to a beta blocker responds to neostigmine (Pratila and Pratilas 1977).

Reid (1978) discusses the use of the ECG in assessing the clinical electrophysiological properties of the antidysrhythmic drugs and its use in assessing the value of the drugs in the management of cardiac dysrhythmias.

Antidysrythmic drugs have been comprehensively reviewed by Carson *et al.* (1979).

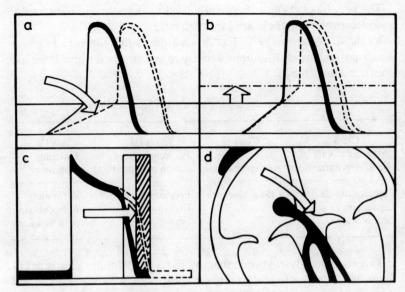

Fig. 68. Targets in antidysrhythmic therapy: (a) Slowing rate of rise of spontaneous diastolic depolarization; (b) increasing the threshold potential; (c) prolonging the refractory period; (d) blocking a re-entry circuit in the AV node.

5

THE ECG DURING ANAESTHESIA AND SURGERY

The ECG provides the best simple monitor of the condition of the patient's heart during surgery. Hence its frequent use in the operating theatre.

Within the operating theatre the ECG differs in two important aspects from one recorded in the out-patient clinic or ward. The first of these is the greater opportunity for the introduction of artefacts, and the second is the rapidly changing pattern of the recorded signal due to the effects of anaesthesia and surgery.

During anaesthesia and surgery, conditions are frequently changing; there are alterations in the concentration of the anaesthetic agents administered, manoeuvres such as intubation, alterations in posture, respiration, temperature, blood pressure and pulse rate.

Few ECG studies have been conducted under regional analgesia. Only general anaesthesia will be considered here.

ECG CHANGES PECULIAR TO THE THEATRE SUITE

Artefacts

AC interference or 'hum'. This may be produced in endoscopes in situ, e.g. bronchoscopes and cystoscopes when using mains reduction, by inadequate earthing of the ECG, or by inadequate earthing of other electrical apparatus, e.g. an electric blanket in use on the operating table. Interference produced by 50-cycle a.c. is illustrated in figure 56.

Diathermy current. The high frequency vibrations of the diathermy current completely obliterate the cardiac potentials and such interference is illustrated in figure 69. Efficient filters make it possible to eliminate the effect of diathermy.

Metal objects.   Large steel retractors, metal suckers and scissors in contact with the patient may induce static charges or may short-circuit the cardiac potentials resulting in deflections which simulate extrasystoles (figure 70).

Muscle tremor.   This may follow an injection of suxamethonium or be associated with shivering during the induction of hypothermia or during the subsequent rewarming. It may simulate fibrillary and ectopic atrial contractions which completely obscure the P waves, and is illustrated in figure 52.

Diaphragmatic contractions.   These may be produced during a period of hiccups and during periods of tachypnoea associated with trichlorethylene or halothane anaesthesia and cause deflections which may resemble atrial ectopic beats (figure 71).

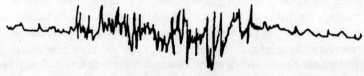

Fig. 69. Diathermy effect.

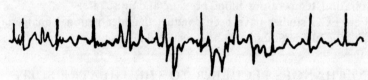

Fig. 70. Artefacts produced by retractors, metal suckers and scissors.

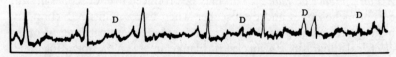

Fig. 71. Deflections produced by diaphragmatic contractions (D).

Pump oxygenator.   An unusual artefact has been reported by Cannard *et al* (1960) where a sine wave was produced by electrochemical potentials generated within the oxygenator (figure 72).

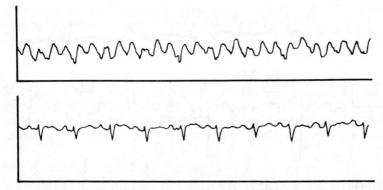

Fig. 72. Upper tracing: sine wave artefact produced by pump oxygenator. Lower tracing: the true ECG picture.

Pacemaker. When a pacemaker is in use the ECG pattern is complicated by the pacemaker pulses. This is illustrated in figure 73.

Identification of artefacts. There is no single technique by which artefact can be recognized and eliminated. Very low or very high voltage in the recorded signal and abnormal wave forms different from the patient's preoperative tracing should cause the anaesthetist to suspect artefact.

Intubation, endotracheal suction and extubation

In the author's view significant ECG changes during intubation, endotracheal suction and extubation are rare in the absence of hypoxia, electrolyte imbalance, CO_2 retention or cardiac disease, but minor dysrhythmias are commonly seen. Amongst the changes observed are: tachycardia, bradycardia, atrial, nodal and ventricular extrasystoles, atrial fibrillation, nodal rhythm, heart block, decrease in the height of the T wave and depression of the ST segment (Rollason and Hough 1957a, Noble and Derrick 1959, Johnstone and Nisbet 1961, Hutchison 1967, Dottori *et al* 1970, Mandappa 1971, Prys-Roberts *et al* 1971, Bertrand *et al* 1971, Saarnivaara and Kentala 1977).

Cardiac arrest on rare occasions has been associated with these manoeuvres. In the severely burned patient the risk is greater (Fleming *et al* 1960, Bush *et al* 1962). The manoeuvres often produce a marked pressor response (Rollason and Hough 1957a). This response may be

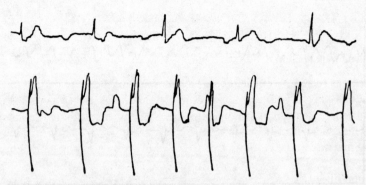

Fig. 73. Upper tracing: the true ECG picture. Lower tracing: artefact produced by an intraventricular stimulator (pacemaker).

prevented by the alpha blocker phentolamine which has an inotropic and antidysrhythmic action of its own (Gould 1969). The response may also be blocked by the use of neurolept-anaesthesia using droperidol and fentanyl in substantial dosage as induction agents (Rollason and Emslie 1972). Practolol in a dose of 0·4 mg/kg is also effective.

Posture and controlled respiration

Changing the patient's posture, e.g. into the lateral or Trendelenburg positions may result in axis deviation. The employment of controlled respiration with deep inflation made possible by complete curarization or deep anaesthesia may also result in axis deviation and this is illustrated in figure 74.

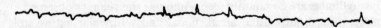

Fig. 74. Changes in electrical axis produced by controlled respiration.

Controlled respiration to the point of hyperventilation producing a PCO_2 level in the region of 15 to 20 mmHg may provoke ECG changes of an ischaemic type and Lamb *et al* (1958) have reported both supraventricular and ventricular dysrhythmias during controlled respiration or hyperventilation. Hyperventilation may produce a transient inversion of the T wave.

ECG CHANGES ASSOCIATED WITH SPECIAL ANAES-THETIC TECHNIQUES

Induced hypotension

Success is related to efficient continuous monitoring of the patient and the ECG plays a vital role in detecting dysrhythmias and in some cases myocardial ischaemia. Changes in the ST segment and the T wave provide evidence of possible myocardial ischaemia and call for immediate increase in the blood pressure (figure 75). The ganglionic blocking drugs *per se* do not appear to produce changes in the ECG nor does sodium nitroprusside (Simpson *et al* 1976).

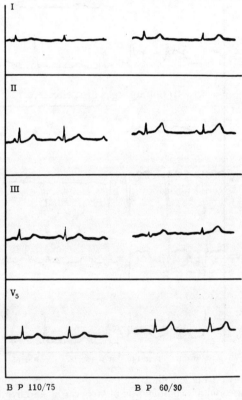

B P 110/75   B P 60/30

Fig. 75. Elevation of the ST segment and increase in the height of the T wave during the hypotensive phase.

It has been shown that ECG changes are significantly higher and their magnitude greater when the hypotension is associated with tachycardia (Rollason and Hough 1959, 1960; see figure 76). This suggests the use of agents such as halothane and techniques such as epidural and spinal which are associated with a bradycardia.

The incidence of ST and T wave changes is greater when the rate of fall of blood pressure is rapid (Rollason 1965, Rollason and Hough 1969). See figures 77 and 78.

In order to correct the tachycardia sometimes associated with hypotensive anaesthesia a cardioselective beta blocker may be used.

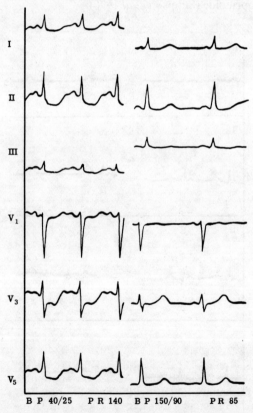

Fig. 76. Tracings on the left illustrate the gross ST depression which can be associated with a combination of tachycardia and hypotension. Tracings on the right illustrate that these changes are reversible when the BP is raised and the PR slowed.

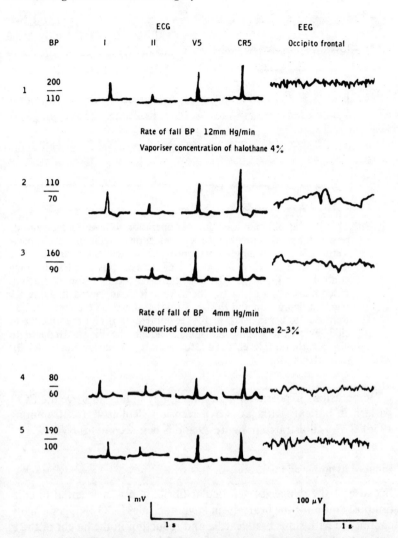

Fig. 77. In this 84-year-old man the BP initially falls rapidly (12 mmHg/min) and ST depression and delta rhythm become apparent. Halothane is then discontinued and the BP allowed to rise. This is subsequently lowered gradually (4 mmHg/min) but to a much lower level, yet the signs of ischaemia previously seen do not appear. It will be observed that the ECG changes are not apparent in lead II, the one commonly used by investigators, and stresses the importance of not relying on a single lead.

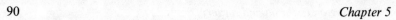

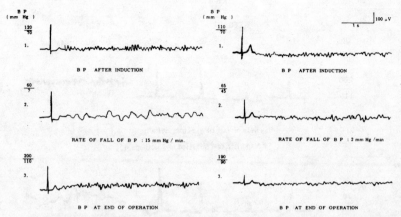

Fig. 78. This 80-year-old man was found at operation to have an oedematous retropubic space, apparently due to infection (tracing on left). Prostatectomy was accordingly postponed and subsequently carried out 2 months later (tracing on right). This patient thus acted as his own control. The ECG (lead II) and the EEG (occipitofrontal) tracings differ markedly on the two occasions. It is suggested that the ST segment depression and the delta rhythm noted on the first occasion were due to a rapid fall in BP (15 mmHg/min) and the absence of changes on the second occasion, although the BP was reduced to virtually the same level, was due to the more gradual lowering of the BP (2 mmHg/min).

On occasions hypotensive anaesthesia may in fact improve the ECG pattern in patients with gross hypertension (Rollason and Cumming 1956). This is illustrated in figure 79 and is best seen in lead V5.

Induced hypothermia

Because of the danger of ventricular fibrillation it is essential to continuously monitor the heart during hypothermia. ECG changes usually commence with sinus bradycardia and reduction in the height of the P wave. As the temperature drops the QRS interval gradually lengthens followed by lengthening and depression of the ST segment and T wave changes (figure 80). At lower temperatures PQRST complex tends to become unrecognizable and dysrhythmias develop. These take the form of atrial fibrillation, extrasystoles and runs of ventricular tachycardia which end in ventricular fibrillation. It should, however, be stressed that ventricular fibrillation in hypothermia can occur without any previous

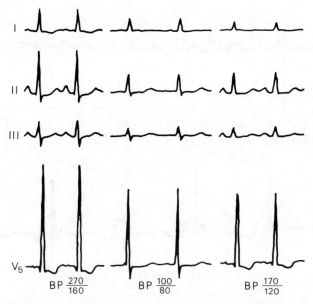

Fig. 79. L.V. 'strain' pattern disappears when BP falls.

changes in the ECG pattern. Figure 81 shows a characteristic wave in the ECG tracing, the so-called J deflection first described by Osborn (1953) and seen during hypothermia but this is of no clinical significance.

When moderate hypothermia is used the customary limit of cooling is 28°C to 30°C.

In profound hypothermia, the patient is usually a child or neonate with a congenital cardiac defect. The patient is on an extracorporeal pump and is cooled to 14°C or below and the ECG undergoes changes characteristic of cooling, bradycardia being followed by varying degrees of heart block, culminating in ventricular fibrillation or asystole. Atrial fibrillation is not as a rule observed. Occasionally the atria continue to beat at a slow rate in the presence of ventricular fibrillation.

The ECG during this ventricular fibrillation often shows a characteristic wave form of groups of complexes see figure 82. When this pattern has become well established, the ECG carries a good prognosis as defibrillation often occurs spontaneously on rewarming. During the period of circulatory arrest there is a state of suspended animation, cardiac and respiratory functions are in abeyance and the ECG, unless

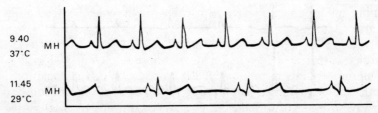

Fig. 80. Upper tracing is normal. Lower tracing shows prolongation of the PR, QRS and ST intervals during induced hypothermia.

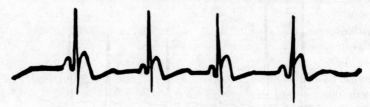

Fig. 81. The Osborn wave.

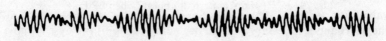

Fig. 82. Ventricular fibrillation pattern during profound hypothermia illustrating groups of complexes.

the heart is fibrillating, is isoelectric. Often fibrillation is not seen at any time during the operation.

The ECG changes associated with accidental hypothermia have been reviewed by Coniam (1979).

ECG CHANGES ASSOCIATED WITH SURGICAL PROCEDURES

Cardiac surgery

Continuous accurate ECG monitoring is essential during cardiac surgery. Remote limb leads have to be used and some units prefer needle to surface electrodes in order to maintain a high quality of recording.

ECG changes should be assessed in conjunction with changes in arterial and central venous pressure which reflect changes in cardiac output and in conjunction with any change in the colour or tone of the heart.

During induction of anaesthesia dysrhythmias may seriously reduce cardiac output in a group of patients whose output may already be compromised by ischaemic or valvular heart disease or a combination of both. The dysrhythmias may be triggered off by hypoxia occasioned by airway problems or stimuli such as laryngoscopy and tracheal intubation under light anaesthesia or by pre-existing electrolyte imbalance, notably hypokalaemia. They can largely be avoided by ensuring that the patient is normokalaemic, by heavy opiate premedication and by a smooth induction of anaesthesia based on narcotics. Should dangerous dysrhythmias such as ventricular tachycardia occur there should be no delay in instituting cardiopulmonary by-pass.

In the seriously ill patient it may be necessary to resort to femoro-femoral by-pass prior to induction of anaesthesia, the lines having been inserted under local anaesthesia.

During surgery, when the heart is exposed, surgical manipulation, insertion of sutures and the placement of clamps tend to produce a variety of dysrhythmias. ECG changes occurring during a simple mitral valvotomy are illustrated in figure 83. Treatment is to stop stimulating the heart and if necessary shift an occluding clamp. If the dysrhythmia persists and is associated with a drop in cardiac output it may be necessary to go on to cardiopulmonary by-pass.

A variety of methods are used to achieve the quiet bloodless field necessary for accurate speedy surgery. Examples are:

1. Aortic cross clamping.
2. Ischaemic arrest at normothermia or moderate hypothermia. (The sequence of ECG changes associated with ischaemic arrest at normothermia are illustrated in figure 84.)
3. Cross clamping and electrical fibrillation of the heart.

There is currently a move away from methods which are associated with anoxic myocardial damage to techniques designed to provide maximal myocardial preservation. In order to reduce metabolism during the period of circulatory arrest after aortic cross clamping a cardioplegic solution with a high potassium concentration at 4°C is injected rapidly into the aortic root. All electrical activity ceases within two minutes and this state is maintained by keeping the septal temperature at between 10°C and 15°C by irrigating the surface of the heart with ice cold saline and employing systemic hypothermia to 25°C. Any return of

1. Tracing taken just prior
   to opening the thoracic
   cavity.

2. After occluding clamp
   applied. Note acute injury
   pattern simulating anterior
   myocardial infarction.

3. Ventricular fibrillation
   followed.

4. Position of occluding
   clamp was shifted and
   ventricular fibrillation ceased.

5. Temporary right B B B
   during closure of the
   atrial appendage

6. During closure of the
   thoracic cavity the E C G
   returned essentially to normal
   and remained so.

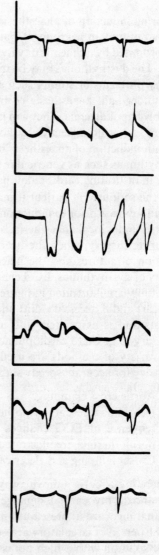

Fig. 83. Lead I taken in all tracings.

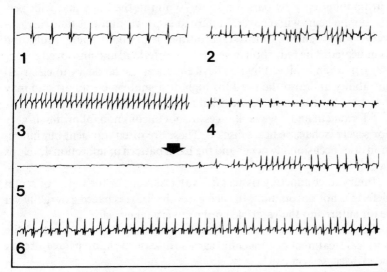

Fig. 84. ECG tracings during operation for closure of VSD and refashioning of pulmonary valve in a child. (1) Prior to application of aortic clamp; (2) shortly after application of clamp; (3) 2 min later; (4) 9 min after application of clamp; (5) to left of arrow: tracing when clamp has been in situ for 24 min; to right of arrow: tracing immediately after removal of clamp; (6) continuation of tracing (5).

myocardial activity is suppressed by a further bolus of cardioplegic solution. On releasing the aortic clamp and reperfusing, the heart either spontaneously resumes sinus rhythm or is readily converted from ventricular fibrillation by a d.c. countershock.

Provided the acid-base and electrolyte (particularly potassium) status are normal few dysrhythmias are seen coming off by-pass provided the left ventricle is efficient. If the left ventricle is only able to provide a low cardiac output dysrhythmias are more common and more dangerous. A low systemic blood pressure and a high end diastolic left ventricular pressure lead to reduced coronary artery perfusion and inotropic drugs needed to improve output are, with the exception of dopamine, arrhythmogenic. Ventricular tachycardia and ventricular fibrillation are treated by d.c. countershock. If they recur, myocardial irritability can be suppressed by lignocaine 1 mg per kg injected as a bolus intravenously.

If it proves impossible to achieve a stable rhythm and a reasonable cardiac output with inotropic support it may be necessary to return to

cardiopulmonary by-pass for 15 to 20 min in the hope that with perfusion the heart will recover. Failure to improve after this time carries a
very poor prognosis. At this stage, intra-aortic balloon counterpulsation
is indicated. The reduction in ventricular afterload and improved coronary perfusion achieved by this device reduces the tendency to electrical
instability and also the need for high dose inotropic support and may
buy time for continued myocardial recovery.

ST segment and T wave changes are not uncommon following surgery
for severe ischaemic heart disease. These are often transient but infarction does occasionally occur and the ECG pattern of infarction develops
later.

Injury to conducting tissue after valve surgery or the repair of septal
defects is not uncommon. In such cases the heart is paced externally via
leads sutured to the ventricle until recovery takes place.

ECG changes associated with profound hypothermia used in the
surgical treatment of congenital cardiac disease in children have already
been discussed on p. 91.

The operation for insertion of a pacemaker in Stoke-Adams disease is
an increasingly common procedure. A permanent pacemaker is im-
planted in the chest wall after control of the heart rate has been achieved
by a temporary pacemaker. This procedure must be carried out with
continuous ECG monitoring to ensure that any problem in switching
from one pacemaker to the other is immediately seen and the minimal
voltage required to pace is easily identified.

The use of diathermy is precluded during this procedure because of
interference with the pacemaker and the risk of inducing ventricular
fibrillation.

The appearance of a paced ECG is shown in figure 73.

In the postoperative period following successful surgery dysrhythmias are rare. Tachyarrhythmias are treated with digitalis and recurring
frequent ventricular ectopics by a slow infusion of lignocaine or practolol if the cardiac output is good. Those patients on inotropic support are
at highest risk of developing ventricular tachycardia and sudden ventricular fibrillation.

During intraoperative epicardial hypothermia the T wave is usually
inverted (Fink *et al* 1977). Other intraoperative situations where the T
wave may become inverted are as follows:

1. Elevated intramyocardial pressure.
2. Acid base and electrolyte disturbance.

3. Hypotension.
4. Bundle branch block.
5. Digitalis effect.
6. Hyperventilation.

Neurosurgery

For posterior fossa procedures and those operations in the sitting position it is advisable to monitor the ECG continuously as a non-specific warning system (Whitby 1963). The absence of ECG changes does not necessarily indicate an adequate circulation and emphasizes the importance of maintaining spontaneous respiration. Air embolism may produce dysrhythmias and, if large, acute cardiac failure. Runs of ventricular extrasystoles and marked bradycardia with or without idioventricular rhythm are dangerous and the surgeon should be warned immediately. The ECG differentiates between a true bradycardia and alternating ventricular extrasystoles.

In posterior fossa procedures Lewis and Rees (1964) emphasize the importance of not relying on a single ECG lead and recommend the routine use of precordial lead V1 and standard leads I and III. Should air embolism occur the resulting strain on the right ventricle due to acute pulmonary obstruction and myocardial ischaemia may be reflected in these leads as follows:

Lead V1: Right bundle branch block, inversion of the T wave and a tall tented P wave
Leads I and III: S1, Q3, T3 or S1, T3 patterns.

Neurosurgical procedures involving the medulla, pons, and the fifth, ninth and tenth cranial nerves often show ECG changes such as ventricular extrasystoles and nodal bradycardia of sufficient magnitude to require remedial action.

During pneumoencephalography particularly in patients with a pituitary tumour and raised intracranial pressure dysrhythmias are frequent (Vourc'h & Tannières 1978).

In the treatment of congenital hydrocephalus by the establishment of a ventriculovenous shunt, the ECG provides a useful means of locating the tip of the catheter in the mid-atrium. The usual practice is to use the tip of the catheter as an electrode in place of the right-arm electrode and to observe either leads I or II. The catheter electrode is either a metal stillette inserted within the catheter or alternatively the catheter is filled

Standard lead II

Probe: superior vena cava

Probe: high atrium

Probe: mid or low atrium (desired position)

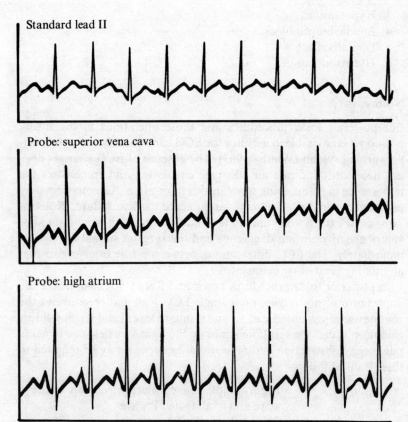
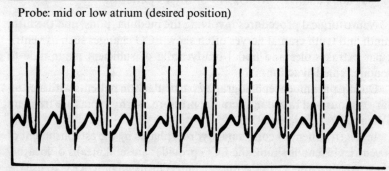

Fig. 85. ECG tracings illustrating intravascular recordings at various positions of the probe tip during a catheter placement.

with 3% saline. The ECG pattern is very sensitive to the exact position of the catheter tip in the heart and no difficulty is found in locating the desired position (Richards and Freeman 1964, Frazer and Galloon 1966). This is illustrated in figure 85.

ECG changes simulating myocardial ischaemia may be produced by cerebral causes. These may be cerebrovascular accidents (Heron and Anderson 1965, Eisalo *et al* 1972) or raised intracranial pressure (Jachuck *et al* 1975).

Renal homotransplantation

Hyperkalaemia is always a risk with these patients and the ECG can be an effective means of monitoring it (Strunin 1966).

The use of stored blood with its high potassium content for transfusion may augment the risk and the appearance of tall tented T waves could indicate the need for the administration of calcium.

Removal of phaeochromocytoma

Before the introduction of alpha and beta blockade this procedure was hazardous due to the release of sympathomimetic amines. ECG monitoring should, however still be used.

Obstetrics

Labour is not a procedure where it is routine to take a maternal ECG. It may be desirable, on occasion, to monitor the maternal ECG for women with a previous cardiac history. It is increasingly common to take fetal ECG's as soon as the cervix dilates sufficiently for a scalp electrode to be introduced. The interpretation of the fetal ECG is in the hands of the obstetrician.

Out-patient surgery

Dentistry represents a branch of out-patient anaesthesia of sufficient importance to consider in Chapter 8.

Most other out-patient anaesthetic techniques also have a light plane of anaesthesia. Few ECG studies have been made but it seems reasonable for the out-patient with an existing dysrhythmia to be monitored during out-patient anaesthesia (Ostroff *et al* 1977).

Exchange transfusion

The need for close acid-base control during exchange transfusion, coupled with the hazard of potassium and citrate intoxication, calls for ECG control during this procedure especially in children.

MINOR PROCEDURES

Cardiac catheterization

During this procedure atrial and ventricular extrasystoles are common. If dangerous dysrhythmias, such as multifocal ventricular extrasystoles, develop the catheter should be immediately withdrawn until the tip lies outside the heart, and the patient should be ventilated with pure oxygen, even though the blood gases at that stage have not been estimated.

Coronary angiography

This should be conducted under continuous ECG control, particularly when hypotension is employed during the injection of the contrast medium.

Ventricular tachycardia requiring intravenous lignocaine or a beta blocker and ventricular bradycardia requiring intravenous atropine may occur.

Some patients undergoing this procedure may have a high pulmonary vascular resistance and equally balanced left-to-right and right-to-left shunting; under these circumstances, the institution of controlled ventilation may result in a sudden fall of arterial oxygen saturation with bradycardia and ECG changes indicative of myocardial ischaemia.

Cardioversion

The d.c. defibrillator used should have a built-in cardioscope. It is customary to time the shock to occur 20 ms after the peak of the R wave.

Endoscopy

Occasional deaths from dysrhythmia or myocardial infarction have followed oesophagoscopy, cystoscopy and sigmoidoscopy (Fletcher *et al* 1968). When cystoscopy is associated with overdistension of the urinary bladder it may precipitate a ventricular tachycardia (Eggers and Baker 1969).

Electroplexy

This, as in the case of endoscopy, is not usually carried out with ECG monitoring, but cardiac asystole may occur during the clonic phase of the convulsion when atropine has not been administered beforehand.

Atropine has been administered intravenously prior to induction with methohexitone or propanidid, followed by suxamethonium and oxygenation. Then the electric shock was administered. Investigation under ECG control has shown that this procedure normally produces no significant ECG changes (Rollason *et al* 1971).

EMERGENCIES IN THE OPERATING THEATRE

Cardiac arrest

This has been discussed in Chapter 6.

For the poor-risk patient continuous ECG monitoring during surgery should reduce the hazard of cardiac arrest. Experience has shown that the following conditions are among those which may on occasion produce cardiac arrest:

1. Endotracheal intubation.
2. Endoscopy, e.g. bronchoscopy, and cystoscopy and sigmoidoscopy in paraplegics with lesions above D6.
3. Ocular surgery due to the oculocardiac reflex (Pöntinen 1966).
4. Denervation of a hypersensitive carotid sinus and the operation of rhytidectomy (Rose *et al* 1976; Chugtai 1977).

Pulmonary embolism

This produces a characteristic series of ECG changes which, in addition to right heart 'strain' (figure 23), include a large P pulmonale in leads II and III, a prominent S wave in lead I, a deep Q wave and inverted T wave in lead III (figure 86).

Transfusion therapy

Some cases of cardiac arrest encountered during anaesthesia appear to be due to massive blood transfusion or to the transfusion of concentrated or fresh frozen plasma. The cause suggested is the increased ratio of potassium to calcium in the venous return to the heart. The anaesthe-

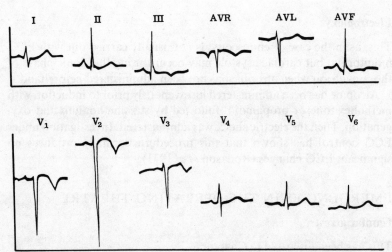

Fig. 86. Acute pulmonary embolism. Note S1, Q3, T3, pattern, right axis deviation and T wave inversion and raised ST segments in leads V1 and V2 and P pulmonale.

tist when supervising one of these transfusions should have the benefit of continuous ECG control and the danger signs are tall tented T waves and prolonged QT intervals. These signs may be reversed by injecting 10% calcium gluconate or chloride slowly intravenously *pari passu* with the blood or plasma but into a different vein. However, except in by-pass open cardiac procedures and exchange transfusion in children, it may not be necessary to administer exogenous calcium (Howland *et al* 1976). The development of gross ischaemic ECG changes or a dangerous dysrhythmia should lead the anaesthetist to suspect air embolism.

The massive transfusion of refrigerated blood may produce cardiac arrest (Boyan and Howland 1961) and a blood warmer should be used.

ECG changes may on occasion be associated with transfusions other than those of blood and plasma.

6

THE ECG IN INTENSIVE CARE
AND CARDIAC ARREST

An intensive care unit should be ready to accept all patients needing the continuous support of a vital function or who are liable to do so at short notice. Conditions calling for intensive care include myocardial infarction, extensive burns, patients undergoing renal dialysis and all conditions requiring artificial ventilation. The latter is the main concern of the anaesthetist.

Those patients whose condition on leaving the operating theatre give grounds for concern should be referred to the intensive care unit.

The prompt recognition of a dysrhythmia and skilful treatment may determine the success of therapy.

Cardiac arrest is more serious when it occurs outside the intensive care unit but this chapter seems an appropriate place to consider this emergency.

THE ECG IN INTENSIVE CARE UNITS

In intensive care units, to facilitate supervision, it is convenient to display physiological parameters for each patient at a central position and where possible to give automatic warning of serious changes in the condition of a patient. No special difficulties occur in producing a central monitoring station except the possibility that data may be ascribed to the wrong patient. The development of automatic warning systems is much more complex because of the need to distinguish between true signals and artefacts and also to decide when a warning should be given. Automatic warning from the ECG is usually restricted to the detection of dysrhythmias and to major changes in pulse rate. The detection usually depends on measurement of the R–R interval and the width of the QRS complex.

103

COMPUTERS

The advent of the silicon chip microprocessor means that the use of computers for patient monitoring and control becomes more feasible; undoubtedly major developments can be expected in the near future. It is necessary to distinguish between this application and the widespread references in the literature to the use of computers for the routine analysis of ordinary clinical ECGs.

The leads used for patient monitoring must be chosen with a view to obtaining a significant ECG tracing and also providing as little inconvenience as possible both to the patient and to the examination of the chest. Electrodes are usually placed on the chest and they will give a tracing approximating to lead II. The electrodes chosen must remain efficient *in situ* for prolonged periods (see Chapter 9).

SIGNIFICANT ECG CHANGES

In modern practice, intensive care has been divided into specialist units. The anaesthetist is mainly concerned with the Respiratory Unit. In other units the interpretation of the ECG will be in the hands of the appropriate specialist.

In the Respiratory Unit the signs of clinical significance are dysrhythmias and changes in the P, T and U waves (Stoddart 1975).

All dysrhythmias may be premonitory signs of ventricular fibrillation and should be regarded seriously but an occasional supraventricular ectopic beat may be of no significance.

Bradycardia may be associated with hypoxia which if undetected may have disastrous results. A cause may be tracheobronchial suction.

A peaked P wave (P pulmonale) may be associated with respiratory failure and indicating the need for IPPV. Too early weaning from the ventilator may be manifest by the reappearance of P pulmonale.

A tall tented T wave or a prominent U wave may suggest electrolyte imbalance which is common in sick patients.

RESPIRATORY CONDITIONS

Status asthmaticus

A right heart strain pattern may develop. This can be reversed by IPPV, bronchodilators and cortisone.

Chest injuries

The ECG may give evidence of cardiac injuries which would otherwise be undetected. This is particularly true of thoracic trauma (Schick *et al* 1977).

Head injuries

When ECG abnormalities are seen these may be due to cerebral causes; already discussed under Neurosurgery (see Chapter 5).

Tetanus

Hypotension may be associated with the onset of myocarditis with characteristic tachycardia, AV block and prolongation of the PR and QT intervals. Hypertension may be associated with ventricular dysrhythmias which respond favourably to treatment with propranolol, bethanidine and anticoagulant therapy (Prys-Roberts *et al* 1969).

In neonatal tetanus ECG changes such as complete bundle branch block may be due to inadequate ventilation (Smythe 1963).

Poisoning

The ECG will monitor the progress of therapy. Treatment for dysrhythmias normally successful may be unavailing in the poisoned patient (Worthley 1974). Poisoning is often produced by overdoses of therapeutic drugs; for many of these drugs there are reports of ECG changes corresponding to normal clinical doses. The large number of these drugs make it impossible to give details for them all. Some are associated with a bundle branch block pattern.

Carbon monoxide poisoning is frequently seen. Its ECG pattern has a characteristic low voltage and ventricular dysrhythmias. These rapidly improve with hyperbaric oxygen therapy.

CARDIAC ARREST

ECG signs of cardiac arrest

When the patient is already being monitored the ECG pattern will

change to one of those usually exhibited at the moment of cardiac arrest.
These are:

1. Ventricular fibrillation.
2. Asystole.
3. Ventricular tachycardia.
4. Ventricular tachyarrhythmia.
5. Complete AV dissociation.
6. Sinus rhythm.

The most usual patterns are ventricular fibrillation and asystole. In
the neonate ventricular fibrillation is unusual. A normal sinus rhythm
may occasionally occur reflecting the uselessness of the ECG as an
indicator of haemodynamic events.

Monitoring the treatment of cardiac arrest

As soon as practicable the ECG should be connected to the patient,
although with modern Cardio/Pak units the paddles of the defibrillator
can be used as electrodes to monitor the ECG.

Precordial thumping

This is an important first-aid measure (Rollason 1978). It will not
usually be monitored by the ECG. When it is, there may be ECG
tracings which appear to suggest success which only reflect electrical
activity (Skaaland 1972). When successful the patient soon returns to
sinus rhythm (see figures 67 and 87).

Electrical defibrillation

Heart action may return or it may remain absent after electrical defibrillation. If it returns the ECG may show the following (figure 88):

1. Normal sinus rhythm.
2. Sinus or nodal bradycardia requiring atropine or isoprenaline.
3. Supraventricular tachycardia requiring electroversion with a
   synchronized shock.
4. Atrial fibrillation or atrial flutter requiring the same therapy as (3)
   above.

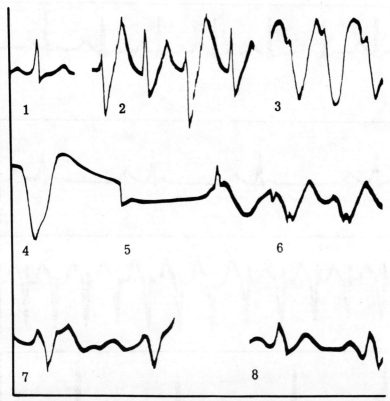

Fig. 87. A case of cardiac arrest occurring during anaesthesia and surgery. Lead II taken in all tracings. (1) Normal ECG; (2) multifocal ventricular extrasystoles; (3) ventricular fibrillation; (4) massage contraction; (5) complex initiated by the heart; (6) intraventricular conduction defect; (7) conduction defect less marked; (8) ECG at the end of the operation.

5. Complete heart block requiring isoprenaline or an artificial pacemaker of the demand type.

If the heart action does not return after electrical defibrillation the ECG may show the following (figure 89):

1. Persistent ventricular fibrillation requiring a cardioselective beta blocker and a higher energy level shock (400 J).
2. Ventricular tachycardia requiring a cardioselective beta blocker and a synchronized shock.

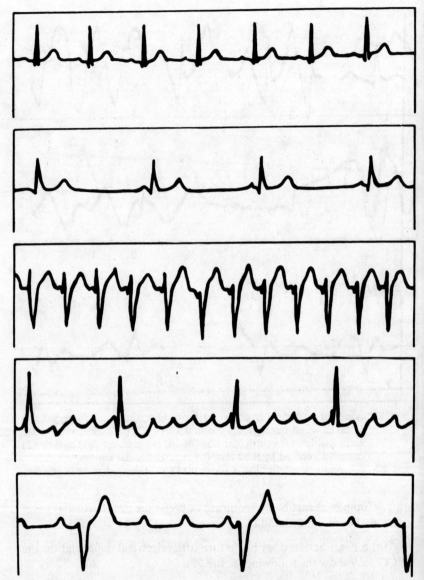

Fig. 88. If heart action returns after electrical defibrillation the ECG may show the patterns illustrated. From above down they are: (1) sinus rhythm; (2) sinus or nodal bradycardia; (3) supraventricular tachycardia; (4) atrial fibrillation or flutter; (5) complete heart block.

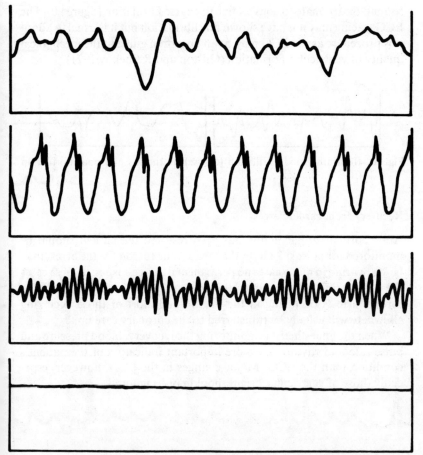

Fig. 89. If heart action does not return after defibrillation the ECG may show the following patterns. From above down they are: (1) persistent or recurrent VF; (2) ventricular tachycardia; (3) ventricular tachyarrythmia; (4) asystole.

3. Ventricular tachyarrhythmia requiring the same therapy as (2) above.
4. Asystole requiring isoprenaline or artificial pacing if it persists.

Cardiac stimulants and the correction of acidosis

If defibrillation fails the next step is to administer cardiac stimulants and sodium bicarbonate to convert fine to coarse fibrillation (figure 90). The ECG tracing may not have shown fine fibrillation but it is usual to adopt this procedure as the ECG may be an uncertain guide to the mechanical quality of ventricular fibrillation (Gilston and Resnekov 1971).

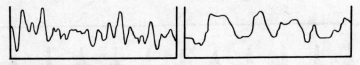

Fig. 90. Illustrates good fibrillation (coarse) on the left and poor fibrillation (fine) on the right.

Recovery from cardiac arrest

After normal cardiac action has been restored the patient should be monitored for at least 24 h. In the theatre, the reason for the arrest may be known and in many cases no permanent damage ensues; in these cases the monitoring will be under the control of the anaesthetist. Other cardiac arrests occurring in the theatre and most of those occurring elsewhere will usually be transferred to the coronary care unit.

When the anaesthetist is monitoring the recovery, blood pressure and pulse rate and rhythm are more important indicators of the patient's condition than the ECG. Major changes in the ECG, however, especially those of ventricular origin should not be ignored.

THE ECG IN ANAESTHETIC RESEARCH

In research, the anaesthetist has two distinct aims, firstly, the study of the physiological effects associated with both anaesthetic agents and drugs used in anaesthesia and, secondly, the improvement of anaesthetic techniques for the benefit of both patient and surgeon.

The ECG studies the electrical activity of the heart and there is no definite correlation between the ECG and heart function. Hence the first question to consider is what can be deduced from the electrocardiogram.

INFORMATION AVAILABLE FROM THE ECG

Typical patterns occurring in abnormal ECGs have been presented in Chapter 3. During anaesthetic procedures the preexisting ECG pattern may change and may simulate one of the abnormal ECGs. The interpretation of the changes needs caution, as marked ECG changes can occur without the corresponding physiological changes; unfortunately, the reverse is also true. The following changes are likely to be seen, however, during anaesthetic procedures.

Heart rate changes.   The ECG usually monitors heart rate efficiently and also gives an indication of the relative lengths of systole and diastole.

Onset of 'ECG myocardial ischaemia'.   The typical pattern of myocardial ischaemia may develop and is illustrated in figures 27 and 76.

The electrical pattern is known to occur only for differential ischaemia, namely, when the magnitude varies in different parts of the myocardium; equally the pattern is not always correlated with other signs of myocardial ischaemia. However, in the circumstances of anaesthesia,

111

the onset of ST depression and T wave inversion can reasonably be considered indications of insufficient oxygenation of the heart.

Development of 'ECG cor pulmonale'.   This shows up as a pattern of right axis deviation, right ventricular 'strain', right bundle branch block, a prominent S wave in lead I and a large Q wave and inverted T wave in lead III (figure 86). This development can usually be taken to suggest a pulmonary embolism. If this is severe the pattern will change to that of cardiac arrest.

Ventricular fibrillation.   This pattern is quite clear and will quickly be confirmed by other indications (figure 33).

Ventricular standstill.   The absence of a QRS complex, even though P waves may be present, means that the heart has gone into asystole.

Electrolyte imbalance.   The ECG can be a sensitive indicator of those changes associated with electrolyte imbalance (figures 62 and 65).

Development of heart 'strain' patterns.   This is associated with characteristic ST and T wave changes (figures 22 and 23) and bundle branch block (figures 48 and 49) is often present as well.

Dysrhythmias.   The main dysrhythmias seen in the ECG are described in Chapter 3. These occur frequently under anaesthetic conditions but seem to be difficult to interpret in terms of risk to the patient.

ANIMAL EXPERIMENTS

The ECG changes discussed above show that they cannot always be related to changes in the heart. The simplicity of ECG measurements makes them attractive and it is obviously useful to do experiments under conditions which permit their correlation with other measurements. In the patient, other interests exist besides research and hence it is valuable to do experiments on animals where the research can be carried through to its logical conclusions.

The use of animal experiments is twofold: first, to persist in a technique producing ECG changes until serious consequences not detectable by other means manifest themselves. This shows that the ECG changes obtained are a useful warning and that it is indeed desirable to take steps to reverse them in clinical usage, Bennett and Eltringham

(1977) used rabbits to study cardiac arrest produced by fenfluramine. In studying hypotensive anaesthesia, Rollason (1965) used the dog in order to be able to examine the ECG changes when hypotension caused myocardial ischaemia of such a magnitude that death ensued (figures 91(a) and (b)). Similarly Stewart *et al* (1965) wishing to examine extreme

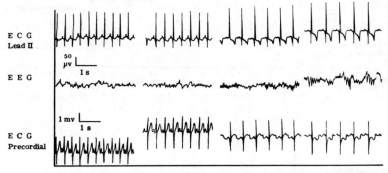

Fig. 91 (a). ECG changes illustrated in lead II and precordial lead and EEG changes (occipitofrontal lead) during increasing normovolaemic hypotension in a dog produced by halothane and IPPR. Other parameters simultaneously recorded include renal blood flow (electromagnetic technique), arterial and central venous pressure illustrated in figures 92(a) and (b). The six tracings were taken on a Devices 8-channel recorder.

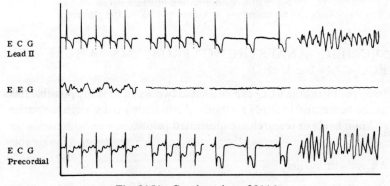

Fig. 91(b). Continuation of 91(a).

acidosis used bull calves. Secondly, by using other measurements of heart parameters it may be seen what actual heart changes, if any, correlate with the ECG changes (figures 92(a) and (b)).

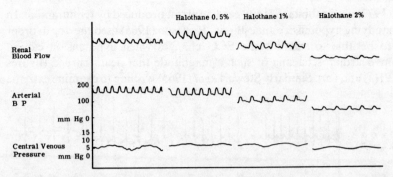

Fig. 92(a). Renal blood flow, and arterial and central venous pressure recorded
simultaneously with parameters illustrated in figure 91(a) and (b).

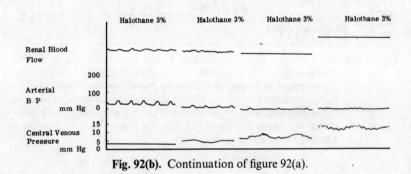

Fig. 92(b). Continuation of figure 92(a).

SPECIFIC ANAESTHETIC PROBLEMS WHERE THE ECG CAN BE USED

In all problems the ECG can be used in two ways: to study possible risks
to the heart; and to study methods of combating risks when they arise.

Main fields of research are illustrated below.

Anaesthetic agents

One of the earliest ECG investigations during anaesthesia was that of
Hill (1932a,b) on multifocal ventricular tachycardia during chloroform
anaesthesia. It has become normal to investigate the use of new anaesthetic agents by ECG studies, e.g. the examination of halothane by
Johnstone and Nisbet (1961). Not only have such studies shown the

potential hazards of anaesthetic agents but they have been extended to demonstrate methods of either eliminating or treating them.

The ECG is also useful for studying anaesthetic agents other than those producing general anaesthesia. For example, Kennedy *et al* (1965) and Kerr (1976) have used it in a study of intravenous regional analgesia using lignocaine and prilocaine.

Drugs used during anaesthesia

The range of drugs used between initial premedication and the recovery room is extensive. All of them are administered for specific purposes and all of them may affect the heart, either in their own right or in association with the anaesthetic agent. Many investigations have been reported of drug activity, and it is not possible to review them all. Reisner and Lippmann (1975) for example, have shown the danger of adrenaline injections during halothane and enflurane anaesthesia, and Johnstone *et al* (1978) have compared the cardiovascular effects of tubocurarine when used with thiopentone or ketamine.

Stimulation effects

The stimulation of the heart produced by endoscopy, oculocardiac reflex etc., causes ECG changes and these may be used to study its magnitude and the efficiency of techniques designed to overcome the consequences. Jenkins (1975) has investigated dysrhythmias during bronchoscopy and Pandit and Pandit (1965) have investigated the control of the oculocardiac reflex with gallamine.

Rollason and Hough (1957a) showed that many of the changes in the QRS complex seen during endotracheal intubation were in fact axis rotation and this shows the value of using a simultaneous two-channel recorder in ECG research (Rollason and Hough 1957b).

Posture

It has been suggested that postural changes may be dangerous during hypotensive anaesthesia and that postural changes in the immediate postoperative period may be particularly hazardous. Whereas these changes may be more significant for the brain, the ECG offers a method of monitoring the heart during postural changes. Posture has been mentioned in the ECG literature but no major investigations seem to have been reported.

Respiration

Under anaesthesia, CO_2 retention becomes a problem and so a major research topic in the study of respiration. Black et al (1959) used an ECG to study cardiac rhythm during halothane anaesthesia when hypercarbia was present; they found that atrioventricular nodal rhythm, ventricular extrasystoles and multifocal ventricular tachycardia were associated with hypercarbia. Hence it is possible to check the efficiency of any ventilation system during halothane anaesthesia by examining the ECG (Eikard and Skovsted 1975).

Hypotensive anaesthesia

Among the major risks of this technique is myocardial ischaemia if the hypotension becomes too great. The ECG provides one of the best simple monitors for this, and so has played a large part in research investigations on the safe use of hypotensive anaesthesia (Simpson et al 1976). One of the controversies about this technique is whether it is likely to increase or decrease the risk of anaesthesia in patients with a previous history of hypertension or coronary disease. The ECG has been used to investigate cardiac changes in such patients (Rollason et al 1964).

Specific surgical techniques

The dangers of cardiac dysrhythmia during anaesthesia may, in certain cases, be more specific to the surgery than the anaesthetic procedure. The ECG can be used to investigate these risks. Whitby (1963), for instance, has compared ECG changes during posterior fossa operations with other neurosurgical procedures. Again, Kaufman (1965) has shown that cardiac dysrhythmia is liable to occur at the moment of extraction during dental surgery under general anaesthesia. An interesting feature of this report is that this original observation was made whilst doing routine ECG monitoring on bad-risk cardiac patients.

Electrolyte imbalance

The ECG is one of the simplest methods of following changes in acid-base balance. Marshall (1962) has used the ECG to illustrate the ill-effects found in cases of massive blood transfusion due to excess potassium. Electrolyte disturbances have also been investigated by Fisch (1973). Johnston (1976) has demonstrated the direct opposition of ketamine and verapamil for the calcium ion.

8

THE ECG IN DENTAL ANAESTHESIA

Over a long period dental anaesthesia was confined either to a local anaesthetic or to 'gas' usually administered by the dentist himself. Then the field of dental anaesthesia began to widen rapidly and has now become a significant branch of contemporary anaesthesia. Yet 'death in the dental chair' still continues to be a problem. Such a rare event—about 1 in 300 000 out-patients (Tomlin 1974)—is difficult to investigate. In trying to make dental anaesthesia safer the idea has developed that relatively minor dysrhythmias can be used as an indication of the safety of dental anaesthesia; the fewer the dysrhythmias the safer the anaesthetic.

TECHNICAL PROBLEMS OF MONITORING THE ECG DURING DENTAL SURGERY

The average duration of dental procedures is short and so it must be possible to connect and disconnect the patient quickly from the ECG machine if the dental surgeon is not to be kept waiting. This makes radiotelemetry the ideal technique (see chapter 9).

Dental ECG investigations are mainly for research and this makes it desirable to keep a permanent record. Dysrhythmias are the main changes and to follow these closely demands a complete record of the ECG throughout the entire procedure. On the grounds of economy this makes tape-recording the method of choice. The tape can be analysed, wiped and re-used.

It is usual to use a single lead and the most popular choices are leads I and II.

118

ANAESTHETIC TECHNIQUES

ECG investigations have been undertaken for most techniques of dental anaesthesia and most anaesthetic agents. The significant ECG changes seen during dental anaesthesia are dysrhythmias.

Local analgesia

While widely used in dentistry it is rarely considered worthy of ECG investigation. Some work has been done using adrenaline and noradrenaline as the vasoconstrictor (Williams *et al* 1963, Hughes *et al* 1966). These investigations were chiefly concerned with the effect of these vasoconstrictors on the heart; a more recent vasoconstrictor used in dentistry, felypressin (Octapressin) does not affect the heart. A comparative study including local analgesia has been made by Ostroff *et al* (1977).

Intravenous techniques

The 'ultra light minimal increment technique' has been investigated for methohexitone and propanidid (Rollason and Dundas 1970) and for althesin (Rollason *et al* 1974). The main ECG change was a sinus tachycardia.

Inhalational techniques

ECG studies have been most frequently made during these procedures. Rollason and Dundas (1970) have studied inhalational techniques alone but these techniques have been more frequently studied in combination with an intravenous induction with or without intubation (Thomas *et al* 1978, Alexander and Murtagh 1979).

DYSRHYTHMIAS

These are mainly ventricular. The precise incidence depends on the specific anaesthetic technique and this makes it difficult to summarize the literature. Most investigators compare two or more techniques but in general few major dysrhythmias are seen. Some of the author's results are shown in Table 3; these figures are fairly typical of the results reported by others. Intubation is a cause of additional dysrhythmias.

Table 3. Incidence of dysrhythmias in relation to anaesthetic technique in dental patients.

Group	Anaesthetic technique	No. of cases	Average age (years)	Average duration of procedure (min)	Incidence of ECG dysrhythmias (%)		
					Major	Minor	Total
I	i.v. only	314	27·7	6·2	0·3	2·5	2·8
II	N₂O/O₂/halothane via nose piece	202	23·6	5·8	1·5	17·2	18·7
III	Marrett N₂O/O₂/ halothane via face piece	201	27·4	7·6	4·0	11·4	15·4
IV	N₂O/O₂/halothane via nasotracheal tube	204	34·2	26·8	4·9	21·1	26·0

The increase in the total percentage of dysrhythmias from 2·8% to 18·7% is statistically significant ($P < 0.001$) and the increase from 18·7% to 26·0% is also significant ($P < 0.05$).

THE AUTONOMIC NERVOUS SYSTEM

Emotional stress

Taggart *et al* (1976) investigated emotional stress in a group of fit young nurses attending for routine restorative dental procedures under local analgesia with felypressin as the vasoconstrictor. They found a significant fall in heart rate whilst the patient sat in the dental chair prior to the administration of the local anaesthetic. They conclude that marked parasympathetic activity overrode an enhanced sympathetic response—the so called 'forgotten vagus'.

Exodontia

Kaufman (1965) observed dysrhythmias at the time of extraction of teeth during general anaesthesia. Plowman *et al* (1974) showed that the blockade of the jaw with local anaesthetic agents reduced the incidence of these dysrhythmias. These observations have been repeated for many different anaesthetic techniques and it would appear that many of the dysrhythmias seen in dental anaesthesia are due to the stimulation of the autonomic system. The lightness of the plane of anaesthesia used for dentistry enables the surgical stimuli to reach the autonomic system via the trigeminal nerve.

The dysrhythmias are usually minor and so it is difficult to justify the routine use of a deeper plane of anaesthesia.

ROUTINE MONITORING IN DENTAL SURGERY

Research investigations do not suggest that it is desirable to monitor the ECG of every patient undergoing dental anaesthesia. On occasions where a patient has a cardiac history it is useful to monitor the ECG continuously to give early warning of impending cardiac crisis. It may also be worth monitoring those patients who are excessively nervous as this predisposes them to cardiac dysrhythmia; and those who, although they give no cardiac history, have preoperative ventricular ectopic beats.

The beta blockers practolol and metoprolol have proved effective in both the prevention and treatment of dysrhythmias occurring during dental anaesthesia (Rollason and Hall 1973, Rollason and Russell 1979). See figures 61(a), (b) and (c).

9

ELECTROCARDIOGRAPHIC EQUIPMENT
SUITABLE FOR USE BY THE
ANAESTHETIST

It is difficult to make any recommendations for the type of equipment required by the anaesthetist as the purposes and the resources in both money and personnel differ so widely. Valuable research has been done with the simplest equipment when the anaesthetist has had sufficient enthusiasm. It seems best, therefore, to discuss the ECG machines (electrocardiographs) in general and then to consider what features are particularly desirable for routine and research use.

ELECTROCARDIOGRAPHIC MACHINES

Since Einthoven's original string galvanometer, the application of electronics has at the same time made the equipment simpler to use and more difficult to understand. The underlying principles behind the measurement of the ECG are considered in an elementary fashion in Appendix I.

The purpose of an ECG machine is to detect the changes of potential produced by the heart between two electrodes placed at suitable positions on the patient and to make these changes visible to the observer. The potential to be detected is quite small, of the order of 1 mV, and the changes occur rapidly (the QRS complex only lasts from 0·05 to 0·10 s). The potential is superimposed on the skin current which is a d.c. potential. This may be as great as 20 mV, and varies slowly with time. The machine must separate the potential due to the heart from the skin current, amplify, and then record the result (the electrocardiogram) in either a permanent or a temporary form.

It is the recorder which is of greatest significance to the anaesthetist. If it is to follow faithfully the shape of the potential between the electrodes, it must be capable of travelling several centimetres in 0·01 s and be capable of making rapid changes in direction without lag. Mathematicians have shown that it is possible to estimate the way in which a recorder will follow a complicated voltage pattern from the way in which it responds to simple sine waves of different frequencies. To follow the potential wave from the heart, the ECG machine should have a flat response from about 0·05 Hz to 100 Hz.

ECG monitor

The ECG is displayed on a cathode ray tube. The older simpler machines have a long afterglow screen with the tracing gradually fading and being overwritten with the next tracing. Modern monitors have a memory system and no longer use a long persistence screen. Instead data from the memory is displayed. The memory element is adapted every 4 or 8 s and so a continuous uniformly bright trace is produced. The memory provides two other useful functions. The first is a freeze which holds a particular tracing for an indefinite period. The second is to provide two tracings on the oscilloscope. The upper one is continuously updated but is transferred as a whole every 4 or 8 s to the lower tracing. This process is called cascade and it is usually the lower picture which is frozen. This enables a comparison to be made of the present ECG picture with that of a fixed reference time.

Cardio-Miniscopes have built-in tripod electrodes which can be directly applied to the precordium of the patient and an immediate ECG tracing observed on the miniscope. It is useful to have one in surgical out-patient theatres when the patient presents with an irregular pulse or develops one during anaesthesia.

The Visicard-Recorder interprets a cardioscope and recorder allowing documentation of an ECG on a record strip after having seen an interesting tracing on the screen.

Most monitors incorporate the heart rate meter and may be part of a larger monitoring system enabling other parameters to be followed. The heart rate meter usually incorporates alarms to indicate serious bradycardia or tachycardia.

In the ECG monitor filters can be incorporated to remove undesired frequencies from the signal. In the theatre, the diathermy machine provides a high frequency signal and a suitable filter reduces this to negligible proportions. In research applications it is important to look closely at the frequency response because it may be desired to record fine details of the ECG which demands a response to high frequencies.

Schick *et al* (1977) were interested in notches in the QRS complex which many ECG machines would fail to record.

ECG recorders

The cardiologist uses a multichannel recorder. Single channel recorders are widely used both for emergency observations and in the theatre. The difficulty with all direct writing recorders is the high velocity and acceleration needed if the pen is to satisfactorily record the details of the ECG pattern. A heated stylus is commonly employed as the pen but a recorder using an ink jet may be more satisfactory for recording the fine details of the tracing.

Magnetic recording

The use of a tape-recorder enables the complete ECG tracing throughout a lengthy procedure to be stored. This enables data to be analysed after the event and so ensures that the ECG can be studied during periods when changes might have been expected. Compared with direct writers the cost of storing ECGs is almost negligible. This is especially true when the tape is wiped and reused.

Choice of ECG equipment

For routine use in the theatre a single-channel ECG monitor usually suffices. It should contain internal filtration designed to eliminate the effects of diathermy. A direct writer will be an advantage as it will enable records to be kept of unusual tracings.

In the ITU equipment is needed both to monitor and to give warning of serious changes in a number of physiological parameters including the ECG. Modern practice builds all this equipment into a single unit and often centralizes it in a central station to cover all the patients under intensive care.

Research can be done with the usual equipment provided in the theatre. Permanent records are almost essential. It is a distinct advantage to have equipment that enables two or more leads to be recorded simultaneously. Some research involves the simultaneous recording of the ECG and arterial pressure or other physiological variables. Before embarking on a major research project it is desirable to consult the hospital physicist to ensure that appropriate equipment is available.

ELECTRODES

Many types of electrode have been used over the years in the attempt to obtain a satisfactory contact with the patient. Ask *et al* (1979) have studied the electrical and mechanical long-term properties of sixteen commercially available electrodes. Although many of these did make a good contact current practice favours two types of electrode.

Disposable electrodes. A sealed packet provides an electrode already coated with electrode jelly. It can be applied to the unprepared skin and gives an excellent contact over a period of days.

Simondsen and Weel Ltd., Series 800 electrodes include types suitable for all age groups, different types of skin resistance, and high humidity situations such as in incubators. They also produce a patient-safe electrode resistance meter to locate a faulty electrode which can then be replaced.

Intek Cardiomat. An ingenious electrode system primarily for use in the theatre is a thin card translucent to X-rays and has three longitudinal strips of aluminium foil on it. Each strip acts as an electrode and the card is placed under the patient. No contact jelly is needed and satisfactory tracings are obtained. This electrode system is basically suitable to monitor dysrhythmias but owing to the uncertainty in its location with respect to the heart will not correspond very well with the standard leads. The cardiomat, although officially designed as disposable, is frequently used more than once (Macnab and Pope 1976). A modification of this is the Roussell Distrode—Back Plate Electrode.

LEADS AND INTERFERENCE

A good tracing depends on a satisfactory path between the patient and the input of the ECG machine. In addition unwanted signals will reach a machine via the same leads. Unwanted signals are usually called interference and the worst enemy is the 50-Hz mains. Interference is reduced by keeping leads short and well screened. The contact between the patient, electrode and the lead, is a place where high impedance can occur leading to a poor tracing; clean surfaces and careful adjustment should eliminate this difficulty. An unsatisfactory earth is often the cause of bad tracings.

126 *Chapter 9*

RADIOTELEMETRY

Radiotelemetry is a technique of taking measurements over a distance
by means of radio. It was first applied to the ECG by Holter (1957). The
development of microelectronics has reduced the size of the transmitter
and its power source to very small dimensions and a correspondingly
small weight. Its use makes it possible to take ECGs during vigorous
exercise and it thus led to research on the ECG performance of athletes.
It has been found to be a very convenient method of monitoring dental
procedures (Rollason and Dundas 1970). The convenience of no leads
suggests it might find wide use in the operating theatre. The layout used
for dental anaesthesia is shown in figures 93(a), (b) and (c).

The use of radio waves means that the frequency must be carefully
chosen so that another radio signal does not interfere at the receiver with
the signal from the transmitter. Again the signal from the transmitter
despite its low power may cause interference in the vicinity. Frequency
bands have been allotted for radiotelemetry and a licence is required in
Great Britain. The British frequency band allocated for medical purposes is 102·2 to 102·4 MHz.

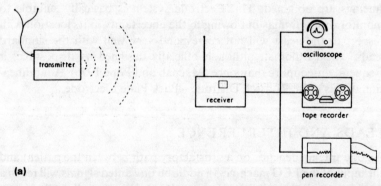

(a)

Fig. 93. Radiotelemetry system. (a) Diagrammatic illustration of the system.
(b, facing page) System currently used. E: AO (American Optical)
electrodes; T: transmitter; R: receiver; M: monitor displaying a two-
trace non-fade ECG with cascade and freeze; alphanumeric heart rate
displaying with alarm limits; DW: direct writer; IRM: instantaneous
heart rate meter; TR:tape recorder. (c, facing page) Tracings produced
by the system compared with that of a conventional direct writer (top
tracing).

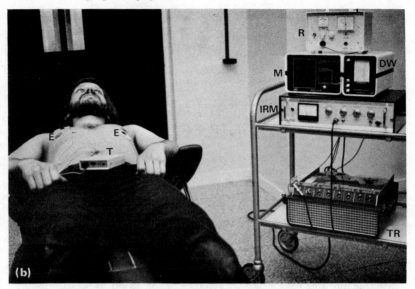

Direct – from ECG machine

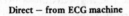

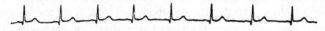

As recorded from receiver

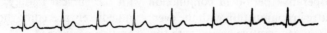

Playback from tape recorder

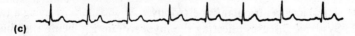

(c)

10

THE VALUE AND LIMITATIONS OF
THE ECG

The ECG provides the anaesthetist with a record of the heart rate and its rhythm, the site and number of the pacemakers, the efficiency of the conducting tissue and the position of the heart. It provides a means of recording fluctuations of autonomic tone produced by the various drugs used by him or his surgical and cardiological colleagues, and is a valuable index of the electrolyte balance of the blood. It is essentially a picture of the site of origin of the stimulus potential, and the speed and direction in which it travels to initiate the myocardial contraction. As the conducting system and the myocardium derive their nutrient from a common blood supply, the coronary arteries, it seems reasonable to assume that any drugs or manoeuvres which produce electrocardiographic evidence of impairment of one may involve impairment of the other (Johnstone 1956). The ECG can be a valuable aid to the anaesthetist preoperatively, during surgery and anaesthesia and in the postoperative period. The ECG changes, however, must be interpreted in the preoperative period in conjunction with the clinical findings, in the theatre in conjunction with the events immediately preceding them, and in the postoperative period with the operation performed.

ECG PREOPERATIVELY

The ECG can elucidate the following conditions:

1. Atrial and ventricular hypertrophy.
2. Systemic diseases affecting the myocardium e.g. acute rheumatic fever.
3. Myocardial infarction.
4. Pericarditis.

5. Dysrhythmias and conduction defects.
6. Electrolyte imbalance.
7. Effects of cardiac drugs.
8. Coronary insufficiency.

ECG DURING ANAESTHESIA AND SURGERY

Here the ECG is valuable:

1. In the evaluation of new agents, drugs and techniques.
2. In the detection of cardiac arrest.
3. As a continuous monitor during: (a) cardiac, vascular and neuro-surgery; (b) removal of a phaeochromocytoma; (c) hypotensive anaesthesia; (d) hypothermia; (e) any type of surgery in the poor risk patient.

The development of the following should be viewed with concern and immediate remedial action taken:

1. Tachycardia above 160 beats per min.
2. Bradycardia below 40 beats per min.
3. Acute cor pulmonale.
4. Multifocal ventricular extrasystoles.
5. Gross ST segment and/or T wave changes and/or inverted U waves.
6. Tall tented T waves with a prolonged QT interval.
7. 'Dying heart' pattern.

It has been suggested (Lown *et al* 1967) that ventricular ectopic beats should be suppressed e.g. by lignocaine, practolol or metoprolol if they have one of these four characteristics: they are of the 'R on T' type; they are of the multifocal variety; there are salvos of two or more; they are sustained in occurrence at a frequency greater than five per minute.

ECG POSTOPERATIVELY

The prompt recognition of a dysrhythmia and its skilful treatment may well determine the success of the recovery from the surgical procedure.

Drugs used to treat an abnormal rhythm should be administered not only under continuous ECG control but under the advice and guidance of a cardiologist.

Atrial, nodal and ventricular extrasystoles which are initiated during a cardiotomy may persist for a day or two into the postoperative period.

The ECG should be checked 24 h postoperatively in patients over 50 years of age with known coronary heart disease, hypertension, diabetes mellitus, peripheral vascular disease or abnormal preoperative ECGs.

LIMITATIONS OF THE ECG

The ECG only portrays the electrical activity of the heart and provides no indication of the strength of myocardial contraction and no record of haemodynamic events. Indeed, it has, on occasion, been known to provide a relatively normal tracing, certainly in a single standard lead, when the heart has ceased to beat effectively as a pump. An illustration of this is shown in figure 94. The patient had clinically been dead for

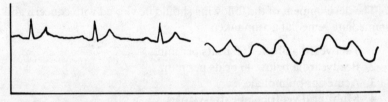

Fig. 94. Tracings on the left: Normal ECG tracing but patient clinically dead. Tracings on the right: taken 30 s later—ventricular fibrillation.

some minutes when the relatively normal tracing was recorded and it was not until the lapse of a further half minute that this tracing changed into one of ventricular fibrillation.

On the other hand, the ECG may, on occasion, show grossly bizarre patterns in the presence of adequate blood pressure. This does not call for panic, but the anaesthetist should ascertain the cause of the abnormal pattern and if possible remove it.

Cardiac dysfunction in the perioperative period has been discussed by Lappas (1977).

Finally it should be stressed that the ECG should be used only as an ancillary aid and the anaesthetist should realize that it is no substitute for keen and constant clinical observation before, during and after surgery. The colour, BP, pulse rate, capillary refill time and pupil size should be frequently checked and take priority over any ECG tracings, except during periods of elective cardiac arrest.

APPENDIX I
BASIC PRINCIPLES OF RECORDING THE ELECTRICAL ACTIVITY OF THE HEART

The electrical activity of the heart produces an approximately cyclical electrical potential at any point on the body's surface. The cycle frequency is the heart rate, and the potential difference between two points on the body surface has a maximum of a few millivolts in the QRS complex. ECGs are the record of the way the potential varies over the entire heart cycle and so the aim of any recorder is to give an undistorted picture of the potential difference over the heart cycle. Thus an ECG machine must detect, amplify and then display and/or record the potential difference as a function of the time.

When an ECG machine has been made, the further question arises as to how truly the pattern obtained represents the actual potential difference produced by the heart between the measuring electrodes. The two most usual limitations are noise and distortion. Noise is the part of the final signal not caused by the heart and can be subdivided into the part entering the system at the electrodes—often called interference—and the part generated inside the machine itself. Distortion is the change in the pattern produced by the imperfection of the machine itself, i.e. the inability to exactly reproduce the input pattern.

Many of the above points apply to the recording of any physiological variable and so a science of medical electronics has developed to produce efficient methods of measuring and recording physiological variables. Few people have the ability to be good in every field and so the average anaesthetist will not wish also to be an electronics engineer. He will wish, however, to use his equipment intelligently and to be able to communicate with the electronics specialist. Although fuller accounts exist (Hill and Dolan 1976), it seems appropriate to give a very simple qualitative account of the principles involved in recording an ECG.

PULSES AND FREQUENCY RESPONSE

In a given lead, one heart beat produces a number of rather irregular shaped pulses of which the most important three are the P wave, QRS complex and T wave. Under normal conditions these pulses repeat for each heart beat. Electronics engineers find it difficult to study the way their circuits respond to pulses but find it relatively easy to study response to sine waves of different frequencies. As a sine wave is a sort of pulse it would be useful if a relation could be found between general pulses and sine waves. The mathematical procedure of Fourier analysis has permitted this to be done and so a pulse can be converted into a frequency spectrum. The precise shape of the pulse determines the amplitudes of the different frequencies but approximate upper and lower frequencies of f'_1 and f'_2 Hz will correspond to a pulse duration of $1/f'_2$ s with fine detail of $1/f'_1$ s. Thus taking the entire heart beat as a single pulse the lower frequency will be about 0·5 Hz and an upper frequency of at least 100 Hz will be needed to recover the fine details of the QRS complex.

BASIC PRINCIPLES OF AMPLIFICATION

The electric power which can be drawn from the heart via ECG electrodes is very tiny—probably less than 10^{-9} watts. This power is insufficient to drive pens or deflect the electron beam of an oscilloscope. Thus some system of amplification has to be used. The input signal is used to regulate the source of power so that an output signal of a more powerful kind is available. Many methods of amplification have been used in the past but today the most common one is the use of solid state electronics in the form of either transistors or integrated circuits.

A complete amplified unit can be represented by figure 95.

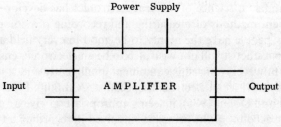

Fig. 95. A complete amplifier unit.

The actual amplifier can take various physical forms but can be regarded as a 'black box' with three pairs of terminals. This is a particularly good description of an integrated circuit which is a tiny chip of metal about 1 mm cube without discrete components. The designer has to know what happens within the 'black box' but the user only needs a specification in terms of the terminals.

The advent of transistors and integrated circuits means that a d.c. voltage of about 10 volts and an almost negligible power consumption is required to drive an amplifier. This means that dry batteries provide a very convenient source of power, but it is quite easy to provide a power pack unit to produce low voltage d.c. from the a.c. mains.

CHARACTERISTICS OF AMPLIFIERS

The four most important characteristics of an amplifier are:

1. The gain

This expresses the degree of amplification produced and is given by:

$$\text{Gain} = \frac{\text{Output power}}{\text{Input power}}.$$

This is frequently in decibels where:

$$\text{Gain} = 10 \ (\log \text{output power} - \log \text{input power}).$$

It is also fairly common to use voltage amplification:

$$\text{Voltage Amplification} = \frac{\text{Output voltage}}{\text{Input voltage}}.$$

If the input and output impedances are the same then the gain is the square of the voltage amplification.

2. Frequency characteristics

For any amplifier the gain varies with the frequency and so it is customary to plot a graph of gain against frequency. Figure 96 shows four common idealized characteristics in (a), (b), (c) and (d).

These amplifiers are characterized by the frequency band f_2 to f_1 which is amplified. For a narrow band amplifier f_2 is nearly equal to f_1 but for

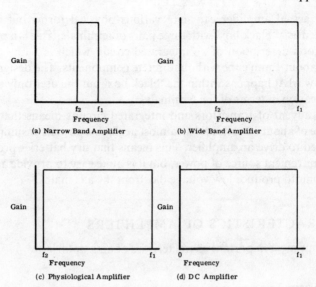

Fig. 96. Four common idealized characteristics: (a) narrow band amplifier; (b) wide band amplifier; (c) physiological amplifier; (d) d.c. amplifier.

the three types of wide band amplifier f_1 is great compared with f_2. For a physiological amplifier f_2 is about 0·01 to 0·1 Hz and f_1 is 100 to 1000 Hz. For a d.c. amplifier the lower limit of frequency is 0 Hz and this provides certain technical difficulties.

The frequency spectrum of a pulse was seen to lie within a frequency range of f'_1 to f'_2. If this frequency range lies within the amplification band f_1 to f_2 of an ideal amplifier, then the pulse will be amplified virtually without distortion; but if the amplification band of the amplifier is smaller than f'_1 to f'_2 Hz the pulse will be distorted.

Real amplifiers do not have ideal characteristics. Thus an actual physiological amplifier will have the characteristics shown in figure 97. Here the frequency is plotted on a logarithmic scale for convenience. By convention the amplifier band f_1 to f_2 is defined as the frequency range within which the gain does not vary by more than ± 3 dB from the 'flat' top of the curve (in the example 140 dB).

In the ordinary ECG machines, the amplifiers are physiological ones. Data transmission over distances is very difficult at these frequencies and so in radiotelemetry and similar systems the pulse is made to

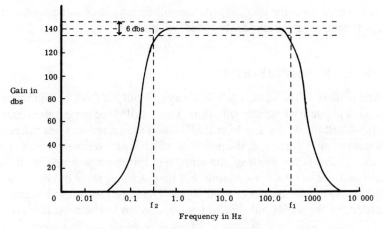

Fig. 97. Characteristics of a physiological amplifier.

modulate a high frequency carrier and the high frequency signals will be amplified in narrow band amplifiers.

3. Input impedance

In electricity, impedance is the ratio of voltage to current for a circuit element. The signal source is feeding power into the input terminals of an amplifier, and so the amplifier looks like an impedance to the source. In practice the impedance is usually a resistance and most amplifiers either have a low input impedance (10 to 1000 ohms) or a high input impedance (100 000 ohms upwards).

In order to get an efficient power transfer the input impedance must be approximately equal to the impedance of the source.

4. Output impedance

The output terminals of an amplifier may be regarded as a source of power to a subsequent stage of output device like a recorder. This source will have an internal impedance which is called the output impedance and is usually a resistance. To get maximum power transfer the output impedance must equal the impedance of the load across the output terminals. If the load is the input of a further amplifier or a cathode ray oscilloscope then the load impedance will be high, but if the load is a loudspeaker or pen recorder the load will be a low impedance.

NOISE IN AMPLIFIERS

Even if there is no input, there is always an output from an amplifier which will fluctuate rapidly with time. This is called the noise output and is produced inside the amplifier itself. Good design reduces but cannot eliminate the noise signal, the power of which is approximately proportional to the band width of the amplifier. For a single amplifier it is difficult to detect the noise output, but then, a single stage of amplification is insufficient to detect a weak signal. Hence further amplification is needed for the signal but this, of course, is given to the noise from the first stage as well. Hence effectively noise is limited to the first stage of an amplifier and the noise generated in this stage can be regarded as a fluctuating noise signal fed into the input terminals along with the signal. The signal to noise ratio expresses the magnitude of the signal compared with the waves. In electrocardiography the signal to noise ratio at the input terminals is large and noise is not an important aspect whereas interference is of great importance.

TYPES OF AMPLIFIERS

Amplifiers can be classified by function as well as frequency characteristics. Most of the amplifiers used inside instruments are concerned with increasing voltage and are called voltage amplifiers. These usually have high input and output impedances. The initial stage of amplification is an important one as the input impedances must be of the same order of magnitude as the impedance of the source of signal and the noise level must be low. It is quite common for the input stage to be in a separate housing from the main amplifier; it is then usually called a pre-amplifier. The output stage of amplification is usually required to deliver power to recorder, loudspeaker etc. and so, in general, needs a low input impedance. Such an amplifier is often called a power amplifier.

RECORDING, STORING AND DISPLAYING THE SIGNAL

The ECG cycle is too short to be followed directly by the human observer and so it is useless to display the output of the amplifier as the movements of a pointer attached to a galvanometer. Thus even display involves an element of storage. Such a display unit is usually called an ECG monitor and presents little difficulty to the user. Display is usually on a cathode ray oscilloscope. The simpler type of monitor uses a screen with a long afterglow so that the trace persists for several seconds. This means that two or three beats can be displayed from left to right across the screen; when the beam is writing the right hand part of the tube, the trace on the left hand side will be fading away and vice versa. This gives a very characteristic look to the screen. Modern monitors make use of memory circuits and a more normal oscilloscope tube without afterglow. The picture is continuously replotted from the data in the memory. The usual tracing covers a period of 4 or 8 s and the memory elements are updated in sequence once per oscilloscope cycle. Many memory monitors have two traces and the data from the upper trace is automatically transferred to the lower end of each oscilloscope cycle—the process is called cascade. The lower trace serves two functions: a simple one of extending the trace slightly into the past and the property 'freeze'. This means that by pressing a button the data on the lower trace remains the same indefinitely; meanwhile, the upper trace displays the current ECG trace.

Recording is usually by the use of some version of pen recorder and storage is on a magnetic tape. Each of these systems introduces a new possibility of error, namely the possibility of both incorrect average speed and fluctuation in the speed of the recording medium.

Pen recorders have a difficult task in that the pen may have to move several centimetres in one hundreth of a second. They are very likely sources of distortion both on account of the limited frequency characteristics and also the non-linear response with frequency.

A tape recorder cannot be used directly to record the output of an ECG because the recorder is not designed to operate at frequencies less than about 50 Hz. So the ECG signal must either be used to modulate a carrier signal or chopped to produce high frequency pulses before it can be fed into a tape recorder. The recorded signal has to go through an appropriate detector system before the signal is converted back to the original ECG. The tape provides a perfectly satisfactory record of the ECG and excellent patterns can be obtained from it. Besides the use of a tape recorder for long-term storage, a short tape loop can be operated as a short-term store. As the tape forms a continuous loop, the ECG record is destroyed after one revolution and replaced by the current ECG; thus the ECG is stored on the tape for the duration of about 1 min. Short term memories of this kind are very useful for dysrhythmia monitors and similar applications.

CONNECTION TO THE PATIENT

The ECG measures the potential difference between two electrodes and so any current drawn from the patient will tend to alter the potential distribution within the patient. This means that the smaller the current drawn by the ECG machine the more correct will be the tracing, i.e. the input impedance of the machine must be very high and is usually several megaohms.

If the input impedance is more than 100 times the impedance of the contact resistance between the electrode and the skin, then the effect of the contact resistance on the ECG tracing will be negligible. This means that provided the electrode–skin resistance is smaller than a few hundred ohms it may be ignored.

The wire joining the electrode to the input terminal will normally have a negligible resistance but can easily be a source of unwanted signals. Any varying electric field in the vicinity of the wire will induce an e.m.f. in the wire and these can easily be at least as large as the ECG signal. This problem is largely overcome by screening the wire. The screen comprises a concentric metal cylinder insulated from the wire and connected to earth. For electrocardiography the use of rigid wires is not feasible and so flexible screen cables have to be used and so both wire and screen take the form of stranded conductors.

UNWANTED SIGNALS

Besides the ECG signal, the electrodes will also detect other e.m.f.s between them. These include potentials produced at the electrodes, other electrical activity of the body and unwanted signals induced in the patient from nearby electrical equipment. The latter is usually described as interference.

Potentials produced at the electrodes will usually be d.c. and so will be rejected by the amplifier. Shivering and muscle tremor will produce electric signals which will appear on the ECG and can be so large that it is impossible to interpret the tracing. Interference caused by an e.m.f. induced in the body is largely eliminated by common mode rejection. At the two electrodes the ECG signal is said to be out of phase whereas an interfering signal will usually be in phase. This means that the potential variation will be in the opposite direction for the ECG signal but in the same direction for the interfering signal at the two electrodes. The right design of the input stage of an amplifier means that theoretically the in-phase signal is rejected and the out-of-phase amplified—common mode rejection. In practice this is not completely achieved but the common mode signal is reduced by about 1000 compared with the wanted signal. If the resistance of the two electrodes differs substantially then common mode rejection will not be so effective. For details of this important topic see Hill (1973).

CALIBRATION

It has become conventional to record ECG patterns so that an input signal of 1 mV is recorded as a deflection of 10 mm; any tracing which does not conform is liable to mislead the cardiologist as to the state of the electrical activity of the patient. Every ECG machine has means of adjusting the amplifier gain so that the correct amplification is achieved.

An internal source of 1 mV is provided and a calibration of the machine can be made using this source. The calibration of an ECG machine should frequently be checked.

STANDARDIZATION

If an ECG tracing is to be useful the machine must satisfy many criteria. It is unreasonable to expect the user to be sufficiently skilled to evaluate a machine himself. Thus a standard specification is desirable and then manufacturers can certify that their machine satisfies this specification. Such a specification is provided by the American Heart Association (Kossmann *et al* 1967).

APPENDIX II.
DYSRHYTHMIAS OCCURRING DURING ANAESTHESIA

TYPE	CAUSES	TREATMENT
EXTRASYSTOLES a. Atrial b. Nodal c. Ventricular	Hypoxia CO_2 retention Anaesthetic agents especially chloroform in the presence of adrenaline Atropine Digitalis Metabolic derangement Hypothermia Intubation Cardiac catheterization Coronary angiography Cardiac surgery	Remove offending stimulus Ensure adequate oxygen- ation and CO_2 elimin- ation Correct electrolyte im- balance and metabolic acidosis Raise BP and temperature if indicated Drugs: lignocaine, practolol or metoprolol Terminate surgery
TACHYCARDIA a. Supraventricular b. Ventricular	Hypoxia Haemorrhage Drugs: adrenaline, chlorpromazine, gallamine, atropine Catheter in the heart Surgical manipulation of the heart	Remove offending stimulus Restore depleted blood volume Carotid sinus and eyeball pressure Drugs: vasopressors, digitalis (if not due to digitalis toxicity), lignocaine, practolol or metoprolol Terminate surgery

TYPE	CAUSES	TREATMENT
BRADYCARDIA	Irritant anaesthetic vapours Drugs: neostigmine, suxamethonium, digitalis, vasopressors C_3H_6, $CHCl_3$ and halothane Overdistension of the lungs in controlled respiration Surgical stimulation of the vagus Traction on extrinsic muscles of eye	Remove offending stimulus IV atropine
AV BLOCK	Cardiac surgery e.g. mitral valvotomy Repair of VSD	Remove offending stimulus e.g. suture involving the bundle of His, finger or valvulotome in the heart, clamp occluding a coronary artery Insert internal pacemaker if AV block is complete and will not respond to drugs such as atropine and isoprenaline
VENTRICULAR FIBRILLATION	Hypoxia Infarction Hypothermia	Adequate oxygenation and CO_2 elimination Cardiac massage Restore myocardial tone with adrenaline or 10% $CaCl_2$ and give 4·2% sodium bicarbonate and 50% glucose Raise temperature, if low Electrically defibrillate

REFERENCES

Adgey A.A.J. & Webb S.W. (1979) The treatment of ventricular arrhythmias in acute myocardial infarction. *Brit. J. Hosp. Med.* **21,** 356

Allan C.M., Cullen W.G. & Gullies D.M.M. (1961) Ventricular fibrillation in a burned boy. *Canadian M.A.J.* **85,** 432

Alexander J.P. & Murtagh J.G. (1979) Arrhythmia during oral surgery: Fascicular blocks in the cardiac-conducting system. *Brit. J. Anaesth.* **51,** 149

Annotation (1970) Ectopic beats. *Lancet* **1,** 603

Ask P., Öberg P.A., Odman S., Tenlund T. & Skogh M. (1979) ECG Electrodes: A study of electrical and mechanical long-term properties. *Acta Anaesth. Scand.* **23,** 189

Averill K.H. & Lamb L.E. (1959 Less commonly recognised action of atropine on cardiac rhythm. *Amer. J. Med. Sci.* **237,** 304

Baillie T.W. (1969a) Ventricular ectopic activity following intravenous ergometrine. *Anaesthesia* **24,** 253

Baillie T.W. (1969b) The influence of ergometrine on the initiation of cardiac impulse. *J. Obstet. Gynaec. Brit. Cwlth.* **76,** 34

Baraka A. (1968) Safe reversal (1). Atropine followed by neostigmine. An electrocardiographic study. *Brit. J. Anaesth.* **40,** 27

Benaim M.E. (1972) Asystole after verapamil. *Brit. Med. J.* **2,** 169

Bennett J.A. & Eltringham R.J. (1977) Possible dangers of anaesthesia in patients receiving fenfluramine. *Anaesthesia,* **32,** 8

Bertrand C.A., Steiner N.V., Jameson G.A. & Lopez M. (1971) Disturbances of cardiac rhythm during anaesthesia and surgery. *J.A.M.A.* **216,** 1615

Bigger J. T. Jr & Goldreyer B.N. (1970) Mechanism of supraventricular tachycardia. *Circulation* **42,** 673

Black G.W., Linde H.W., Dripps R.D. & Price H.L. (1959) Circulatory changes accompanying respiratory acidosis during halothane anaesthesia in man. *Brit. J. Anaesth.* **31,** 238

Bourdillon P.J. (1977) ECG lead systems. *Brit. J. Clin. Equip.* **2,** 285

Boyan C.P. & Howland W.S. (1961) Blood temperature. A critical factor in massive transfusion. *Anesthesiology* **22,** 559

Brichard G. & Zimmerman P.E. (1970) Verapamil in cardiac dysrhythmias during anaesthesia. *Brit. J. Anaesth.* **42,** 1005

Bromage P.R. (1967) Extradural analgesia for pain relief. *Brit. J. Anaesth.* **39,** 721

References   143

Brown B.R. & Crout J.R. (1968) The sympathomimetic effect of gallamine on the heart. *Anesthesiology* **29**, 179

Büchner Ch., Steim H. & Drägort W. English Edition by Schamroth, L. (1977) *The Cardiac Arrhythmias.* Boehringer, Ingelheim

Burch G.E. & De Pasquale N.P. (1964) *A History of Electrocardiography.* Year Book Medical Publishers, Chicago.

Bush G.H. (1964) The use of muscle relaxants in burnt children. *Anaesthesia* **19**, 231

Campbell D., Forrester A.C., Miller D.C., Hutton I., Kennedy J.A., Lawrie T.D.V., Lorimer A.R. & McCall D. (1971) A preliminary clinical study of CT 1341—a new steroid anaesthetic agent. *Brit. J. Anaesth.* **43**, 14

Carson I.W., Lyons S.M. & Shanks R.G. (1979) Anti-Arrythmic Drugs. *Brit. J. Anaest.* **51**, 659.

Chughtae A.L. (1977) Carotid sinus syncope. *J.A.M.A.* **237**, 2320

Coniam S.W. (1979) Accidental hypothermia. *Anaesthesia* **34**, 250

Davies C.K. (1965) Adrenaline and halothane. *Anaesthesia* **20**, 374

Dawson B., Theye R.A. & Kirklin J.W. (1960) Halothane in open cardiac operations: a technique for use with extracorporeal circulation. *Anesth. and Analg. Curr. Res.* **39**, 59

Deutsch S. & Dalen J.E. (1969) Indications for prophylactic digitalization. *Anesthesiology* **30**, 648

Donaldson R.M. (1979) The treatment of supraventricular arrhythmias. *Brit. J. Hosp. Med.* **21**, 344

Dottori O., Egenberg K.E. & Löf B. Axson (1970) Electrocardiographic changes during nitrous oxide-oxygen-relaxant anaesthesia in cardiac patients. *Brit. J. Anaesth.* **42**, 711

Dubin D. (1971) *Rapid Interpretation of ECGs,* 2nd ed. C.O.V.E.R. Inc. Tampa, Florida

Eikard B. and Skovsted P. (1975) Effects of respiratory acidosis on the arrhythmia threshold during fluroxene and halothane anaesthesia. *Acta Anaesth. Scand.* **19**, 120

Eikard B. & Sorensen B. (1976) Arrhythmias during halothane anaesthesia. (I) The Influence of atropine during induction with intubation *Acta Anaesth. Scand.* **20**, 296

Eikard B. & Andersen J.R. (1977) Arrhythmias during halothane anaesthesia. (II). The influence of atropine. *Acta Anaesth. Scand.* **21**, 245

Eerola R., Pöntinen P.J. & Miettinen P. (1963) Electrocardiographic changes during neurolept-analgesia. *Acta Anaesth. Scand.* **7**, 187

Eggers G.W.N. & Baker J.J. (1969) Ventricular tachycardia due to distension of the urinary bladder. *Anesth. and Analg. Curr. Res.* **48**, 963

Egilmez A. & Dobkin A.B. (1972) Enflurance (Ethrane, compound 347) in man. *Anaesthesia* **27**, 171

Einthoven W. (1903) Die galvanometrische Registrierung des menschlichen Elektrokardiograms. Zugleich eine Beurteilung der Anwendung des Capillar-elektrometers in der Physiologie. *Pflugers Arch. ges. Physiol.* **99**, 472

Eisalo A., Peräsalo J. & Halonen P. I. (1972) Electrocardiographic abnormalities and some laboratory findings in patients with subarachnoid haemorrhage. *Brit. Heart J.* **34**, 217

Falk R.B. Jr, Delinger J.K. & O'Neill M.J. (1977) Changes in the electrocardiogram associated with intra-operative epicardial hypothermia. *Anesthesiology* **46**, 302

Fisch C. (1973) Relation of electrolyte disturbances to cardiac arrhythmias. *Circulation* **47**, 408

Fleming J.F. (1979) *Interpretation of the ECG*. Update Books, London, Fort Lee

Fletcher G.F., Ernest D.L., Shuford W.F. & Wenger N.K. (1968) Electrocardiographic changes during routine sigmoidoscopy. *Archives Int. Med.* **122**, 483

Foëx P. (1977) Beta-adrenergic blockade, arrhythmias and anaesthesia. *Proc. Roy. Soc. Med.* 79, Suppl. 11, p.17

Forbes A.M. (1966) Halothane, adrenaline and cardiac arrest. *Anaesthesia* **21**, 22

Fraser J.G., Ramachandran P.R. & Davis H.S. (1967) Anesthesia and recent myocardial infarction. *J.A.M.A.* **199**, 318

Frazer A.K. & Galloon S. (1966) Intracardiac catheterisation. *Lancet* **2**, 1133

Fukishima K., Fujita T., Fugiwara T., Ooshima H. & Sato, T. (1968) Effect of propranolol on the ventricular arrhythmias induced by hypercarbia during halothane anaesthesia in man. *Brit. J. Anaesth.* **40**, 53

Gilston A. & Resnekov L. (1971) *Cardio-respiratory Resuscitation*. Heinemann, London

Goldman V., Astrom A. & Evers H. (1970) A study of the interaction between a tricyclic antidepressant and some local anaesthetic solutions containing vasoconstrictors. *III Asian Australian Congr. Anaesthesiology* 517

Gordon N.L.M., Smith I. & Swapp G.H. (1972) Cardiac arrhythmias during laparoscopy. *Brit. Med. J.* **1**, 625

Gottlieb, J.D. & Sweet R.B. (1963) The antagonism of curare: the cardiac effect of atropine and neostigmine. *Canad. Anaesth. Soc. J.* **10**, 114

Griffiths H.W.C. (1979) *Lecture on 'Chloroform' to N.E. Scotland Society of Anaesthetists*. Dundee, 5th April

Grogono A.W. (1963) Anaesthesia for atrial defibrillation. Effect of quinidine on muscular relaxation, *Lancet* **2**, 1039

Hampton J.R. (1977) The management of cardiac arrhythmias. *Brit. J. Hosp. Med.* **17**, 160

Hartley A. (1979) Extracardiac factors influencing electrocardiography. *Brit. J. Hosp. Med.* **21**, 328

Hart D.D. & Duthie A.M. (1964) The effect of chloroform and halothane administration on the liver. *Proc. III Congr. Mund. Anaesthesiol.* **2**, 86

Heard J.D. & Strauss A.E. (1918) A report on the electrocardiographic study of two cases of nodal rhythm exhibiting R–P intervals. *Amer. J. Med. Sci.* **155**, 238

Heron J.R. & Anderson E.G. (1965) Concomitant cerebral and cardiac ischaemia. *Lancet* **2**, 405

Hill D.W. & Dolan A.M. (1976) *Intensive Care Instrumentation*. Academic Press, London

Hill I.G.W. (1932a) Cardiac irregularities during chloroform anaesthesia. *Lancet* **1**, 1139

Hill I.G.W. (1932b) The human heart in anaesthesia: an electrocardiographic study. *Edin. Med. J.* **39**, 533

Holter N.J. (1957) Radioelectrocardiography: a new technique for cardiovascular studies. *Ann. N.Y. Acad. Sci.* **65**, 913

Howland W.S., Schweizer O., Jascott D. & Ragasa J. (1976) Factors influencing the ionisation of calcium during major surgical procedures. *Surg. Gynec. Obstet.* **143**, 895

Hudon F. (1961) Methoxyflurane. *Canad. Anaesth. Soc. J.* **8**, 544

Hughes C.L., Leach J.K., Allen R.E. & Lambson G.O. (1966) Cardiac arrhythmias during oral surgery with local anaesthesia. *J. Amer. Dent. Ass.* **73**, 1095

Hutchison B.R. (1967) Electrocardiographic changes in children following extubation. *Med. J. Austr.* **1**, 151

Jachuck S.J., Ramani P.S., Clark F. & Kalbag R.M. (1975) Electrocardiographic abnormalities associated with raised intracranial pressure. *Brit. Med. J.* **1**, 242

Jenkins A.V. (1975) Electrocardiographic findings during bronchoscopy. Use of the Sanders' ventilating attachment. *Anaesthesia* **30**, 548

Johnstone M.W. (1948) *The Effects of General Anaesthetic Agents on Abnormal Hearts. A study of Electrocardiology.* (Thesis) Queens University, Belfast

Johnstone M.W. (1951) Pethidine and general anaesthesia. *Brit. Med. J.* **2**, 943

Johnstone M.W. (1956) Electrocardiography during anaesthesia. *Brit. J. Anaesth* **28**, 579

Johnstone M.W. (1971) Oxprenolol (Trasicor) during halothane anaesthesia in surgical patients. *Brit. J. Anaesth.* **43**, 167

Johnstone M.W. (1976) Cardiovascular effects of ketamine in man. *Anaesthesia* **31**, 873

Johnstone M.W. & Barron P.T. (1968) The cardiovascular effects of propanidid; a study in radiotelemetry. *Anaesthesia* **23**, 180

Johnstone M.W., Mahmoud A.A. & Mrozinski (1978) The cardiovascular effects of tubocurarine in man. *Anaesthesia* **33**, 587

Johnstone M.W. & Nisbet H.I.A. (1961) Ventricular arrhythmia during halothane anaesthesia. *Brit. J. Anaesth.* **33**, 9

Jones R.E., Deutsch S. & Turndof J. (1961) Effects of atropine on cardiac rhythm in conscious anaesthetised man. *Anesthesiology* **22**, 67

Katz R.L. & Epstein R.A. (1968) The interaction of anesthetic agents and adrenergic drugs to produce cardiac arrhythmias. *Anesthesiology* **29**, 763

Katz R.L. & Katz G.J. (1966) Surgical infiltration of pressor drugs and their interaction with volatile anaesthetics. *Brit. J. Anaesth.* **38**, 712

Kaufman L. (1965) Cardiac arrhythmias in dentistry. *Lancet* **2**, 287

Kaufman L. (1966) Cardiac arrhythmias during dental surgery. *Proc. Roy. Soc. Med.* **59**, 731

Kennedy B.R. Duthie A.M., Parbrook G.D. & Carr T.L. (1965) Intravenous regional analgesia: An appraisal. *Brit. Med. J.* **1**, 194

Kerr J.H. (1967) Intravenous regional analgesia (A clinical comparison of lignocaine and prilocaine). *Anaesthesia* **22**, 562

Kilpatrick D. (1978) The ECG in ischaemic heart disease. *Brit. J. Hosp. Med.* **14**, 212

Kossman C.E., Brody D.A., Burch G.E., Hecht H.H., Johnston F.D., Kay C., Lepeschkin E. & Pipberger H.V. (1967) Recommendations for standardisation of leads and of specifications for instruments in electrocardiography and vectorcardiography. *Circulation* **35**, 583

Krikler D.M. (1974) A fresh look at cardiac arrhythmias. *Lancet* **1**, 851

Krikler D.M. & Goodwin J.F. (1975) *Cardiac arrhythmias*. W. B. Saunders, London

Kristoffersen M.B. & Clausen J.P. (1967) Bradycardia and hypotension during cyclopropane anaesthesia caused by hyoscine as premedication. *Brit. J. Anaesth.* **39**, 578

Krumbhaar E.B. (1918) Electrocardiographic observations in toxic goitre. *Amer. J. Med. Sci.* **155**, 175

Kuner J., Enescu V., Utsu F., Boszormenyi E., Berstein J. & Corday E. (1967) Cardiac arrhythmias during anaesthesia. *Dis. Chest.* **52**, 580

Kurtz C.M., Bennett J.H. & Shapiro H.H. (1936) Electrocardiographic studies during surgical anesthesia. *J.A.M.A.* **106**, 434

de Lange J.J. (1963) Cardiac arrest with halothane and adrenaline. *Anaesthesia* **18**, 537

Lappas D.G. (1977) Cardiac dysfunction in the peri-operative period. *Anesthesiology* **47**, 117

Leigh M.D., McCoy D.D., Belton M.K. & Lewis G.B. (1957) Bradycardia following intravenous administration of succynylcholine chloride to infants and children. *Anesthesiology* **18**, 698

Leighton K.M. & Sanders H.D. (1976) Anti-cholinergic premedication *Canad. Anaesth. Soc. J.* **23**, 563

Lepeschkin E., Marchet H., Schroeder G., Wagner R., De Paula E., Silva E. & Roab W. (1960) Effect of epinephrine and norepinephrine on the electrocardiogram of 100 normal subjects. *Am. J. Cardiol.* **47**, 594

Lewis J.N. & Rees G.A.D. (1964) Electrocardiography during posterior fossa operations. *Brit. J. Anaesth.* **36**, 62

Lively B. (1973) Effect of respiration on Parkinson's tremor. *Brit. Med. J.* **1**, 241

Lown, B., Fakhro A.M., Hood W.B. & Thorn G.W. (1967) The coronary care unit. *J.A.M.A.* **199**, 188

Macnab J.A. & Pope R. (1976) Simplified ECG monitoring with an electrode mat. *Brit. Med. J.* **2**, 506

Mandappa J.M. (1971) Arrhythmia frequency during extubation. *Arch. Anaesthesiol. & Resusc.* **1**, 33

McLeskey C.H., McLeod D.S., Hough T.I. & Stallworth J.M. (1978) Prolonged asystole after succinylcholine administration. *Anesthesiology* **49**, 208

Marshall M. (1962) Potassium intoxication from blood and plasma transfusions. *Anaesthesia* **17**, 45

Massumi R.A., Mason D.J., Amsterdam E.A., De Maria A., Miller R.R., Scheinman M.M. & Zelis R. (1972) Ventricular fibrillation and tachycardia after intravenous atropine for treatment of bradycardia. *New Eng. J. Med.* **287**, 336

Matthias J.A., Evans-Prosser C.D.G. & Churchill-Davidson H.C. (1970) The role of the non-depolarizing drugs in the prevention of suxamethonium bradycardia. *Brit. J. Anaesth.* **42**, 609

Matthias J.A. & Payne J.P. (1970) Practolol in the management of cardiac dysrhythmias in patients anaesthetized with halothane. *Brit. J. Pharmacol.* **40,** 572

Mirakhur R.K., Clarke R.S.J., Elliott J. & Dundee J.W. (1978) Atropine and glycopyrronium premedication: A comparison of the effects of cardiac rate and rhythm during induction of anaesthesia. *Anaesthesia* **33,** 906

Mirakhur R.K. (1979) Intravenous administration of glycopyrronium. *Anaesthesia* **34,** 458

Muravchick S., Owens W.D. & Felts J.A. (1979) Glycopyrrolate and cardiac dysrhythmias in geriatric patients after reversal of neuromuscular blockade. *Canad. Anaesth. Soc. J.* **26,** 22

Noble M.J. & Derrick W.S. (1959) Changes in the electrocardiogram during induction of anaesthesia and endotracheal intubation. *Canad. Anaesth. Soc. J.* **6,** 267

Orr D. & Jones I. (1968) Anaesthesia for laryngoscopy. A comparison of the cardiovascular effects of cocaine and lignocaine. *Anaesthesia* **23,** 194

Orton R.H. & Morris K.N. (1959) Deliberate circulatory arrest: the use of halothane and heparin for direct vision intracardiac surgery. *Thorax* **14,** 39

Osborn J.J. (1953) Experimental hypothermia: respiratory and blood pH changes in relation to cardiac function. *Amer. J. Physiol.* **175,** 389

Ostroff L.H., Goldstein B.H., Pennock R.S. & Weiss Jr W.W. (1977) Cardiac dysrhythmias during out-patient general anesthesia: a comparison study. *J. Oral Surg.* **35,** 793

Owitz S., Pratilas V., Pratila M.G. & Dimich I. (1979) Anaesthetic considerations in the prolonged QT interval (LQTS): a case report *Canad. Anaesth. Soc. J.* **26,** 50

Pandit S.K. & Pandit R. (1965) Occulo-cardiac reflex under general anaesthesia and the use of gallamine as a preventive measure. *Ind. J. Anaesth.* **13,** 80

Plowman P.E., Thomas W.J.W. & Thurlow A.C. (1974) Cardiac dysrhythmias during anaesthesia for oral surgery. The effect of local blockade. *Anaesthesia* **29,** 571

Pöntinen P.J. (1966) The importance of the oculo-cardiac reflex during ocular surgery. *Acta Ophthal, København.* Suppl. 86

Pratila M.G. & Pratilas V. (1977) A case of tachydysrhythmia. Refractory to propanolol and responsive to neostigmine. *Anaesthesia* **32,** 1017

Price H.L., Lurie A.A., Jones R.E., Price M.I. & Londe H.W. (1958) Cyclopropane anesthesia: Epinephrine and norepinephrine in initiation of ventricular arrhythmias by carbon dioxide inhalation. *Anesthesiology* **19,** 619

Prys-Roberts C., Corbett J.L., Kerr J.H., Crampton Smith A. & Spalding J.M.K. (1969) Treatment of sympathetic overactivity in tetanus. *Lancet* **1,** 542

Prys-Roberts C., Greene L.T., Meloche R. & Foëx P. (1971) Studies of anaesthesia in relation to hypertension II: Haemodynamic consequences of induction and endotracheal intubation. *Brit. J. Anaesth.* **43,** 531

Reid W.S. (1978) The electrocardiogram in the assessment of the effect of drugs on cardiac arrhythmias. *Brit. J. Pharmacol.* **6,** 473.

Reisner L.S. & Lippmann M., (1975) Ventricular arrhythmias after epinephrine injection in enflurane and in halothane anesthesia. *Anes. & Analg. Curr. Res.* **54,** 468

Robinson J.S. (1967) Hypotension without hypoxia. *Internat. Anesthesiol. Clinics.* **5,** 467

Rollason W.N. (1957) Atropine, neostigmine and sudden deaths. *Anaesthesia* **12**, 364

Rollason W.N. (1964) Halothane and phaeochromocytoma. *Brit. J. Anaesth.* **36**, 251

Rollason W.N. (1965) The monitoring of hypotensive anaesthesia. *Anaesthesia* **20**, 479

Rollason W.N. (1968) Diazepam as an intravenous induction agent for general anaesthesia. In *Diazepam in Anaesthesia,* eds. P. F. Knight & C. G. Burgess, John Wright, Bristol

Rollason W.N. (1970) Cardio-respiratory changes following induction of anaesthesia with diazepam. In *Proc. III Asian and Australasian Congr. Anaesthesiol.* 418. Butterworths, Australia

Rollason W.N. (1978) The management of cardiac arrest—first aid measures. *Update* **17**, 785

Rollason W.N. & Cumming A.R.R. (1956) The electrocardiogram in hypotensive anaesthesia. *Anaesthesia* **11**, 39

Rollason W.N. & Dundas C.R. (1970) Incidence of cardiac arrhythmias during dental anaesthesia. *Excerpta Medica Intern. Congr. Series No. 200 'Progress in Anaesthesiology',* 969

Rollason W.N., Dundas C.R., & Milne R.G. (1964) ECG & EEG changes during hypotensive anaesthesia for 'no catheter' prostatectomy. *Proc. III. Congr. Mund. Anaesthesiol* **1**, 106

Rollason W.N. & Emslie W.I. (1972) A comparison of pancuronium bromide with tubocurarine. *Asian Arch. Anaesthesiol.* **2**, 14

Rollason W.N., Fidler K. & Hough J.M. (1974) Althesin in outpatient dental anaesthesia. *Brit. J. Anaesth.* **46**, 881

Rollason W.N. & Hall D.J. (1973) The prevention and treatment of dysrhythmias during anaesthesia for oral surgery. *Anaesthesia* **28**, 139

Rollason W.N. & Hough J.M. (1957a) Electrocardiographic studies during endotracheal intubation and inflation of the cuff. *Brit. J. Anaesth.* **29**, 363

Rollason W.N. & Hough J.M. (1957b) A possible fallacy in single lead electrocardiography. *Lancet* **2**, 245

Rollason W.N. & Hough J.M. (1958) Thiopentone induction and the electrocardiogram. *Brit. J. Anaesth.* **30**, 50

Rollason W.N. & Hough J.M. (1959) Some electrocardiographic studies during hypotensive anaesthesia. *Brit. J. Anaesth.* **31**, 66

Rollason W.N. & Hough J.M. (1960) A study of hypotensive anaesthesia in the elderly. *Brit. J. Anaesth.* **32**, 276

Rollason W.N. & Hough J.M. (1960) A re-examination of some electrocardiographic studies during hypotensive anaesthesia. *Brit. J. Anaesth.* **41**, 985

Rollason W.N. & Latham J.W. (1963) Anaesthesia for intracranial aneurysms. *Anaesthesia* **18**, 498

Rollason W.N. & Russell J.G. (1979) An evaluation of intravenous metoprolol in the management of dysrhythmias in out-patient dental anaesthesia. Paper submitted for publication to *Anaesthesia.*

Rollason W.N., Sutherland M.S. & Hall D.J. (1971) An evaluation of the effect of methohexitone and propanidid on blood pressure, pulse rate and cardiac arrhythmia during electroconvulsive therapy. *Brit. J. Anaesth.* **43**, 160

Rose E.H., Laub D.R. & Avakoff J. (1976) Cardiac asystole secondary to carotid sinus compression in the face lift operation. *Plastic and Reconstructive Surgery.* **59,** 252

Rosen M. & Roe R.B. (1963) Adrenaline infiltration during halothane anaesthesia. *Brit. J. Anaesth.* **35,** 51

Ryder W. & Townsend D. (1974) Cardiac rhythm in dental anaesthesia: a comparison of five anaesthetic techniques. *Brit. J. Anaesth.* **46,** 760

Saarnivaara L. & Kentala E. (1977) Comparison of electrocardiographic changes during microlaryngoscopy under halothane anaesthesia induced by althesin or thiopentone. *Acta Anaesth. Scand.* **21,** 71

Salem M.R., Ylagan L.B., Angel J.J., Vedam V.S. & Collins V.J. (1970) Reversal of curarization with atropine neostigmine mixture in patients with congenital cardiac disease. *Brit. J. Anaesth.* **42,** 991

Schamroth L. (1976) *An Introduction to Electrocardiography.* Blackwell Scientific Publications, Oxford

Schamroth L. & Chesler E. (1963) Phasic aberrant ventricular conduction. *Brit. Heart J.* **25,** 219

Schamroth L., Krikler D.M. & Garrett C. (1972) Immediate effects of intravenous verapamil in cardiac arrhythmias. *Brit. Med. J.* **1,** 660

Schick T.D., Van der Zee J. & Powers S.R. (1977) Detection of cardiac disturbances following thoracic trauma with high frequency analysis of the electrocardiogram. *Journal of Trauma* **17,** 419

Schlant R.C. & Hurst J.W. (1976) *Advances in Electrocardiography,* Vol. 2. Grune and Stratton, New York

Scott D.B. & Julian D.G. (1972) Observations on cardiac dysrhythmias during laparoscopy. *Brit. Med. J.* **1,** 411

Seuffert G.W. & Urbach K.F. (1967) Influence of thiopental induction on incidence and types of cardiac arrhythmias during cyclopropane anesthesia. *Anesth. and Analg. Curr. Res.* **46,** 267

Shutt L.E. & Bowes J.B. (1979) Atropine and hyoscine. *Anaesthesia* **34,** 476

Simpson P., Bellamy D. & Cole P. (1976) Electrocardiographic studies during hypotensive anaesthesia using sodium nitroprusside. *Anaesthesia* **31,** 1172

Skaaland K. (1972) Effect of chest pounding: electrocardiographic pattern. *Lancet* **1,** 1121

Smythe P.M. (1963) Studies on neonatal tetanus and in pulmonary compliance of the totally relaxed infant. *Brit. Med. J.* **1,** 565

Solway J. & Sadove M.S. (1965) 4-Hydroxybutyrate—a clinical study. *Anesth. and Analg. Curr. Res.* **44,** 532

Sprague D.H. (1977) Paroxysmal supraventricular tachycardia during anesthesia. *Anesthesiology* **46,** 75

Starre van der P.J.A. (1978) Wolff–Parkinson–White syndrome during anesthesia. *Anesthesiology* **48,** 369

Stephen G.W., Davie I.T. & Scott D.B. (1971) Haemodynamic effects of beta receptor blocking drugs during nitrous oxide/halothane anaesthesia. *Brit. J. Anaesth.* **43,** 320

Strunin L. (1966) Some aspects of anaesthesia for renal homotransplantation. *Brit. J. Anaesth.* **38,** 812

Suppan P. (1979) Althesin in Wolff–Parkinson–White syndrome. *Brit. J. Anaesth.* **51,** 69

Taggart P., Hedworth-Witty R., Carruthers M. & Gordon P.D. (1976) Observations on electrocardiogram and plasma catecholamines during dental procedures: the forgotten vagus. *Brit. Med. J.* **2**, 787

Talbot S. (1979) Ventricular arrhythmias. *Brit. J. Hosp. Med.* **20**, 201

Thomas E.T. (1965) The effect of atropine on the pulse. *Anaesthesia* **20**, 340

Thomas V.J.E., Kyriakou K.P. & Thurslow A.C. (1978) Cardiac arrhythmia during out-patient dental anaesthesia: a comparison of controlled ventilation with and without halothane. *Brit. J. Anaesth.* **50**, 1243

Tolmie J.D., Joyce T.H. & Mitchell G.D. (1967) Succinylcholine danger in the burned patient. *Anesthesiology* **28**, 467

Tomlin P.J. (1974) Death in out-patient anaesthetic practice. *Anaesthesia* **29**, 551

Vaughan-Williams L.E.M. (1970) In *Symposium in Cardiac Arrhythmias* eds. E. Sandoc, E. Henstaad-Jensen, and K. H. Olsen, Astra, Sweden, P.449

Vourc'h G. & Tannières M.L. (1978) Cardiac arrhythmia induced by pneumoencephalography. *Brit. J. Anaesth.* **50**, 833

Ward D.E. & Camm A.J. (1979) Atrio-ventricular block. *Brit. J. Hosp. Med.* **21**, 381

Wheller T., Murrills A. & Shelley T. (1970) Measurement of the fetal heart rate during pregnancy by a new electrocardiographic technique. *Brit. J. Obst. Gynae.* **85**, 12

Whitby J.D. (1963) Electrocardiography during posterior fossa operations. *Brit. J. Anaesth.* **35**, 624

Wig J., Bali I.M., Singh R.G., Kataria R.N. & Khattri H.N. (1979) Prolonged Q-T interval syndrome. *Anaesthesia* **34**, 37

Williams R.M., Keyes M., Beeker .D., Williams R.A. & Wasserman F. (1963) Electrocardiographic changes during oral surgical procedures under anesthesia. *Oral Surgery* **16**, 1270

Worthley L.I.G. (1974) Lithium toxicity and refractory cardiac arrhythmia treated with intravenous magnesium. *Anaesthesia and Intensive Care* **2**, 357

Wynands J.E. & Burfoot M.F. (1965) A clinical study of propanidid. (F.B.A. 1420) *Can. Anaesth. Soc. J.* **12**, 587

Youngberg J.A. (1979) Cardiac arrest following treatment of paroxysmal atrial tachycardia with edrophonium. *Anesthesiology* **50**, 234

INDEX

151